GASTRIC SLEEVE COOKBOOK

The Complete Bariatric Diet Guide With Easy and Healthy
Recipes

(Tasty and Instant Recipes, With Small Protein-packed Meals)

Jason Seiler

Published by Sharon Lohan

© **Jason Seiler**

All Rights Reserved

Gastric Sleeve Cookbook: The Complete Bariatric Diet Guide With Easy and Healthy Recipes (Tasty and Instant Recipes, With Small Protein-packed Meals)

ISBN 978-1-990334-83-2

All rights reserved. No part of this guide may be reproduced in any form without permission in writing from the publisher except in the case of brief quotations embodied in critical articles or reviews.

Legal & Disclaimer

The information contained in this book is not designed to replace or take the place of any form of medicine or professional medical advice. The information in this book has been provided for educational and entertainment purposes only.

The information contained in this book has been compiled from sources deemed reliable, and it is accurate to the best of the Author's knowledge; however, the Author cannot guarantee its accuracy and validity and cannot be held liable for any errors or omissions. Changes are periodically made to this book. You must consult your doctor or get professional medical advice before using any of the suggested remedies, techniques, or information in this book.

Table of contents

Part 1

1

Introduction

Undergoing surgery is usually a scary decision, but nowadays, surgeries have turned into something very common. You may often come across various people around you, in your neighborhood, your family, and friends who may undergo different kinds of surgeries. The scary part does not lie in being operated, but what happens once you are operated. The post-surgery period is quite a difficult time in which we have to face our fears of recovering quickly.

Gastric Bariatric Sleeve Surgery is usually performed to cut down your stomach space, so you may consequently eat very less start shedding pounds easily. This surgery is very common worldwide, especially in the United States, as obesity rates are very high in the country. Many individuals perform this surgery so they can lose weight and hence get rid of obesity. The problems arise in the issues that follow the surgery, and many individuals do not feel comfortable in tackling the situations that arise later on. Eating right and healthy to make your body work effectively is very necessary after the surgery.

In this book, you will come across different, amazing, and easy to make on your own recipes that will assist you in tackling all the issues of your body after gastric bariatric surgery. If you have gone through the surgery already or are planning to undergo surgery, this book is a fantastic guide for you. In this book, you will come across the different advantages of undergoing surgery and will learn how this surgery works. This book will make you prepare for the ultimate journey from the very start to the extreme end of the surgery.

In this book, you will learn the different tips and tricks that will help you in recovering quickly from the surgery. This book contains nutritional guidelines and principles that you need to follow so your body gets all the good stuff in order to work perfectly after the surgery. A 30-day meal plan is also added to the book for some of you who are in search of a good diet plan to follow. You can also quickly formulate your own diet plan after reading this book.

This book contains 100 recipes to follow easily containing therapeutic foods such as broths, juices, smoothies, and salads. You will be given recipes that you can easily add to your breakfast, lunch, and dinner timings. In the end, losing weight is not enough, but maintaining your weight is the most important task. You will be given effective guidelines to keep yourself healthy, sound, and motivated throughout the entire journey. A healthy change in your lifestyle is significant for a healthy body, so let us indulge in the world of health and fitness for a better tomorrow.

Chapter 1: Introduction to Gastric Sleeve Bariatric Surgery

All of us dream of becoming healthy and losing weight so we can look smart and attractive. Gastric Sleeve Bariatric surgery is a surgery that is performed to reduce the mass of the stomach in order to lose weight. In the following subsections, you will learn everything related to the surgery in detail.

1.1 What is Gastric Sleeve Bariatric Surgery?

Gastrectomy is a surgical procedure for the removal of some parts of the stomach. Gastric Sleeve Bariatric surgery is a type of gastrectomy. Gastric Sleeve Bariatric Surgery is a prohibitive procedure. It extraordinarily decreases the overall size of your stomach and also constrains the measure of food that can be eaten at once. It does not cause diminished assimilation of supplements or sidestep your digestive organs. In the wake of eating a limited quantity of food, you will feel full rapidly and keep on feeling full for a few hours. Gastric Bariatric surgery may likewise cause abatement in your cravings. Similarly, lessening the stomach's size, gastric sleeve surgery may diminish the measure of the "hunger hormone" delivered by the stomach, which may add to weight reduction after undergoing this methodology.

Gastric Bariatric surgery, otherwise called the sleeve gastrectomy, has proved to be a famous decision for patients looking for brilliant weight reduction in a clear methodology that does not require the support and long haul complication rates of going through a Lap-Band.

Hugely obese people (individuals with a high BMI, i.e., more than 45) have an expanded risk during any medical procedure. What's more? The more extended the time under sedation, the more noteworthy is the hazard. Gastric detour medical procedure can last for more than 2 hours. Duodenal switch medical procedure frequently assumes control in more than 4 hours. That is quite a while to be under sedation. So specialists started separating the method into two phases. The main stage was to lessen the size of the stomach. The subsequent stage would be done a year later after the person loses some weight. The second phase of the method would incorporate bypassing a portion of the digestive tracts to lessen calorie assimilation. About 75% of the stomach is expelled, leaving a tight gastric cylinder or sleeve. Some of the time, the choice to continue with a two-phase approach is made before the medical procedure because of these realized hazard factors. In different patients, the choice to perform sleeve surgery (rather than bypass) is made during the surgical activity. This choice incorporates unreasonably huge liver or broad scar tissue that would make the bypass method excessively long or dangerous.

Some dangers are normal to any laparoscopic method, for example, bleeding, disease, injury or infection to different organs, or the need to change over to an open surgical method. Likewise, there is a little danger of a leak due to the staple line used in the partition of the stomach. These issues are uncommon, and significant intricacies happen less than 1% of the time. In general, the usable dangers related to Gastric sleeve surgery are somewhat higher than those seen with the lap band yet lower than the risks related to bypass.

1.2 Advantages of Gastric Bariatric Sleeve Surgery

Gastric Bariatric Sleeve Surgery is an insignificantly obtrusive medical procedure to decrease the size of the stomach. It is currently the most mainstream weight reduction in medical procedures all around the world. People frequently observe the extraordinary achievement that their loved ones have had with the sleeve surgery and, at that point, need similar outcomes. Patients accomplish substantial weight reduction with a straightforward activity without too much stress. It bodes well that with a little stomach, you will be able to eat less and lose a lot of weight. The sleeve surgery has been seen as substantially more potent than the gastric band surgery. It does not require the arrangement of an outside gadget or needle modifications which the later needs.

Following are some advantages that come alongside this surgery:

- Hauling around unreasonable weight puts a great deal of pressure on your joints, regularly causing incessant agony and joint harm. The noteworthy and supported weight reduction that happens after bariatric medical procedures diminishes the weight on joints and regularly permits individuals to quit utilizing torment prescriptions and appreciate considerably more mobility.
- Accomplishing and supporting a typical weight territory regularly permits individuals with rest apnea to quit utilizing a CPAP machine at sleep time.
- Bariatric medical procedure causes long haul reduction of hard-to-control type 2 diabetes. The aftereffects of this strategy are exceptionally viable for obese or overweight patients with type 2 diabetes, permitting practically all patients to stay liberated from insulin and subordinate prescriptions for about three years post the medical procedure.
- Numerous hefty individuals feel discouraged due to helpless self-perception and social shame. Considerably more young individuals who convey a critical abundance of weight think that it is hard to partake in exercises they may somehow appreciate, prompting social separation and discouragement that lead to depression. Losing this weight can enhance enthusiastic wellbeing in these patients.

- Weight reduction medical procedure can likewise improve fertility conditions during childbearing years.
- Weight reduction medical procedure can mitigate metabolic disorder, pregnancy entanglements, gallbladder ailment, and that is just the beginning.
- Weight reduction medical procedure diminishes an individual's danger of coronary illness, stroke, and peripheral coronary illness. Circulatory strain and cholesterol levels can come back to typical or close to ordinary after the bariatric medical procedure, decreasing these dangers, and improving general prosperity.

The above advantages are very encouraging and can be helpful to related individuals. With heftiness and its related wellbeing inconveniences increasing at an alarming rate in the world, bariatric medical procedure unquestionably speaks to be an incredible asset for giving supported alleviation to overweight individuals.

1.3 Preparing for Gastric Bariatric Surgery

Preparing yourself for any surgery can seem difficult, but this can be quickly done with the help of the following steps that will give the entire good and positive stuff to get yourself ready:
- Smoking and the utilization of tobacco and nicotine items have been demonstrated to significantly expand the danger of complications during and after bariatric medical procedures. It is recommended that patients quit tobacco just as all nicotine items for at least three months before starting pre-medical procedure instructions.
- Start to consider food as a fundamental fuel for your body and focus on how your body responds to the food you are consuming. Increment your attention to outer signs for eating, just as satiation (feeling of fullness) prompts. Eat carefully and abstain from eating while being occupied like

counting at your work area or while staring at the TV. Concentrate on eating gradually, biting completely, truly tasting, and appreciating your food. Work to decrease or wipe out responsive eating when exhausted, drained, stressed, or utilizing food to adapt to feelings.

- If you are not as of now working out, start little and make a reliable physical movement plan that accommodates your capacity. You can do short strolls, seat activities, and little increments in everyday activities that can have any kind of effect. Discover a movement you can appreciate and center around recurrence as opposed to forcing. Progressively develop practice time by including a couple of moments of physical activity daily.

- Start considering what elements have added to your weight and what has been in the method of making changes throughout your life. Consider your availability for change right now. Consider beginning a list or diary of sound and propelling the way of life transforms you are making. Build up an encouraging group of people consisting of constructive and caring individuals. Discover elective methods of adapting to passionate eating. Always remember that making changes in your lifestyle is a procedure that requires time. Take little strides, set reasonable objectives, and always remain positive.

- It is essential not to put on weight while getting ready for the medical procedure. Maintain a strategic distance from the last supper and avoid stuffing your stomach completely.

- Follow the thirst signals that your body gives you. Grown-ups need at any rate 64 ounces of water each day. Distinguish and restrict or dispose of sources of fluid calories, including liquor, pop, juice, caffeinated beverages, and espresso with added sugar or cream. Wipeout stimulated and carbonated drinks from your routine. Quit drinking fluids with your food and hold up 30 minutes after supper before drinking anything.

- Start reading various books, visit different websites, go to a care group and talk with other people who have had medical procedures to get educated about the methods offered, dangers, and changes that will occur in your lifestyle.
- Attempt to eat three ordinary meals and one to two little snacks every day. When arranging suppers, make sure to incorporate breakfast and attempt to abstain from eating inside four hours of sleep. Concentrate on expanding protein; add fresh fruits and vegetables into your meal timings, while diminishing or wiping out high fat and sugar nourishments, just as fast food and other restaurant chains.
- Recording your eating and drinking propensities can reveal important data and help you recognize open doors for development. Utilize various helpful food and fluid trackers.

Preparing yourself can turn out to be quite an easy job if you follow your instincts and the easy instructions mentioned above.

Chapter 2: The Journey through the Process of Before and After the Surgery

The Journey through the process of before and after the surgery can be a very emotionally stressed one. You need to prepare yourself mentally and physically before undergoing any medical treatment on your body. In this chapter, you will come across different subjects that will help you in a successful surgery both mentally and physically as well as tips to recover quickly from the operation.

2.1 Factors to Consider Before Surgery

Before you choose if this surgery is the best decision for you, you have to know some of the realities associated with the procedure. Despite the fact that bariatric medical procedure is sheltered and, for the most part, fruitful in accomplishing weight reduction, but in order to be a decent up-and-comer, you should be set up to manage both physical and emotionally intense issues. Following are some facts that need a little consideration before undergoing the surgery:

- A Bariatric medical procedure is definitely not a cosmetic strategy. We may want to look better in the wake of getting more fit, yet the best explanations behind experiencing this significant medical procedure are to broaden and improve our lives. There's a typical misinterpretation that most patients who have bariatric (weight reduction) medical procedure recapture their weight. Actually, most bariatric medical procedures patients keep up effective weight reduction in the long haul.
- When you get endorsed for the surgery, you will have to manufacture an emotionally supportive network. One of the most important choices you will make is picking your support group. The relatives, companions, colleagues, and

experts in your group must regard and support your decision. You will have to make arrangements for an all-inclusive recuperation. Past assistance with childcare, family unit tasks, and transportation during and after hospitalization, you will require help for acclimating to the adjustments throughout your life and the feelings that go with those changes.

- You should persuade and advocate for yourself. Pushing for yourself implies instructing yourself, arranging, and figuring out how to support yourself. You should be certain beyond a shadow of a doubt this is the best way for you since you will need to persuade others: your family, your primary care physicians, and your insurance company. To undergo the medical procedure, your primary care physician must suggest it. At that point, you should give at any rate a half year of records indicating your weight and your endeavors to get fit. When you have the specialists ready, your clinical protection supplier must approve the installments.

- Effective patients arrive at little objectives and triumph, keeping themselves motivated. Patients who are roused to get thinner and ready to follow diet post-surgery and exercise preceding the weight reduction medical procedure may encounter more prominent degrees of achievement speedily following the strategy and over the long haul. The vast majority do not wind up genuinely fat in a few days. It takes a long time to arrive at that weight, and hence patients ought to show restraint toward the weight reduction method, which will likewise not occur right away.

When considered, the above factors can lead up to a very good start and a brilliant end to the surgical procedure.

2.2 The Process of Surgery and Recovering After

The surgery process can be made easy if you choose a very professional team of health workers for your operation. The procedure of gastric bariatric sleeve surgery is instead a small one, and the stay at the hospital is also very low about two to three days maximum. The team of health workers will help you control or manage the pain that occurs post-surgery when you are off the anesthesia.

The effect of this surgery on the body is a very positive one with very few to no complications at all. The stomach gets smaller in size, and the overall food it can hold is reduced enormously; thus, weight reduction occurs in a great amount. The hormones produced by the stomach also decrease, which consequently causes satiety or feeling of fullness in the body by reducing the appetite of the individual.

The recovery of the patient after the surgical procedure can be achieved quickly if you follow the instructions that your health provider or doctor gives you. Your calorie intake will reduce enormously to about the quarter of your consumption before the surgery. Your incision site should be properly taken care of, try to apply the different medical ointments regularly that your doctor has recommended. You will have to bring changes in your eating habits that will directly change your lifestyle.

2.3 Tips for Recovering quickly from the Surgery

The Gastric bariatric sleeve medical procedure is the start of a significant life change, and numerous variables will decide its drawn-out impacts on your body and your life's quality. While your primary care physician's aptitude is essential to guaranteeing a smooth medical procedure, your outcomes will likewise, at last, rely upon what you do from the beginning to the end of the procedure. It is critical to remain cheerful, solid, and concentrated on recuperating in the following months, paving the way to and following the weight reduction operation. There are a few tips you can use when the medical procedure to augment the consequences of your treatment and move quicker towards recovery. Following are some recovery tips you can easily follow:

- You will have to change your swathes/bandages and calm your pain as you recuperate, so stock up on fundamental clinical supplies in advance. Put your resources into bandage cushions and cotton balls to supplant the ones you get from the medical clinic. Ensure you have warming cushions and agony relievers close by to soothe or mitigate your reactions.
- As you get in shape in the months ahead, your change will make you experience a few sizes in a generally short measure of time. Before you undergo the medical procedure, ensure you have garments in various sizes, yet do not get a totally different closet. Glance through your wardrobe for old things and peruse second hand shops for this change period.
- If, by chance, you eat more than your post-operation gut can deal with, spewing or vomiting is inescapable. This may be painful and uneasy, so it is critical to modify slowly and figure out how to limit your regurgitating dangers. Eat more slowly than expected, giving your cerebrum enough time to get the sign that it is full, and ensure you bite appropriately and eat a large portion of the sum you figure you ought to from the outset. Try not to drink through a straw, eat too many dry types of nourishment, or hurry through different meals. Rather, take as much time as is needed and keep your bits littler than expected.
- Your stomach can no longer hold huge amounts of nutritious food. However, you need your nutrients and minerals like never before. To ensure you mend appropriately and keep

on getting the nutrients you need, have healthful supplements prepared.

- Rather than getting apprehensive about what-if's, arm yourself with exact data about your medical procedure. Find out about the encounters of different patients, and explore the ideal approaches to get ready for your medical procedure. Discussions and online care groups will enable you to realize what is in store; however, they will likewise become your encouraging network as you recuperate.
- Most bariatric specialists require their patients to quit smoking, at any rate, fourteen days before their method. If you have not jettisoned the propensity yet, medical procedure is an extraordinary inspiration to make it perpetual. Smoking hinders your mending time and prompts incalculable other wellbeing confusion. Liquor is likewise an ill-conceived notion for recouping patients, on the grounds that your throat will be sore from intubation.
- After your remedy painkillers run out, you will need anti-inflammatories to decrease the pain and swelling as you keep on recuperating. Ensure that you have over-the-counter pain-relieving drugs at home for when you need them.
- At the point when you wake up, you will need free, delicate apparel that is anything but difficult to put on. Your body will be too sore to even think about squeezing into tight garments, and anything with clasps, zippers, or fastens could bother your lines. Ensure you have a lot of comfortable garments sitting tight for you at home, as well, and wear baggy clothing to work until your lines and irritation are not an issue anymore.
- Ensure your footwear is agreeable and simple to slip on and off as well. You will not have the option to twist down effectively from the outset, so have slip-on shoes prepared to step into.
- Do you have a companion, accomplice, neighbor, or relative who can get you out while you recuperate? Make this game

plan early, and have a reinforcement alternative prepared in the event that something occurs. Indeed, even light family errands might be hard for the main week, so ensure another person is there to help.

You can easily and effectively recover from the surgery if you follow the above instructions carefully.

Chapter 3: Curing the After Effects of Gastric Sleeve Bariatric Surgery through Diet

Improving your diet can have many benefits. While undergoing a surgery, especially the one related to the stomach, a person needs to be extremely cautious regarding his/ her eating habits. The healthier and simpler is consumed; the better will be the results on the body of the individual. So, this chapter will give you all the information you need regarding your eating habits post the gastric bariatric surgery.

3.1 Nutritional Principles and Gastric Sleeve Bariatric Surgery

Weight reduction medical procedure alone cannot make you fit; it is just proposed to give you a kick off on your way to a healthier weight. Following the medical procedure, you should focus on an entirely different way of life approach to get better results. You will need to follow the simple rules to get a better lifestyle:

- As the food is eaten in very small amounts post-surgery so, it is recommended to take different nutritional supplements, i.e., vitamins and minerals.
- Doing an appropriate physical exercise is also recommended by the doctors, so the body does not become stiff.
- Always visit your doctor regularly after a few days. Having routine checkups after the surgery is a must and is always recommended.
- Taking responsibility for your health is very important. You need to be very responsible after surgery and give yourself care and love.

- Always eat small and healthy meals after the surgery.
- Maintain a healthy, sound, and positive environment around yourself. Do not take any unnecessary stress.

There are some nutritional facts and principles that you can easily follow to bring your body into the exact shape that you have dreamed about. These nutritional facts are easy, understandable, and can be implemented quite easily. Following are some nutritional principles:

- Try to maintain a distance from any sugary foods or beverages, including sodas, sweets, alcoholic drinks, always read the nutritional label before taking any food or beverage.
- Try to eat slowly; chewing your food well should be your priority. Try eating your food in 25 to 30 minutes, and to make this effective, you can use a stopwatch.
- Avoid excessive snacking and try to eat three complete meals during the course of a day.
- It is recommended to take approximately 60 ounces of fluid each day. After surgery, it is always advised to avoid dehydration and constipation.
- Smoking and intake of alcoholic beverages are prohibited post-surgery. The lining of the stomach walls are very sensitive to these substances and can cause irritation of any kind.
- It is also recommended not to drink while having your meals as this may harm the stomach lining. When we drink with food, the stomach swells up. This condition may cause harm to your stomach walls, which are very sensitive right after the surgery. Try to stop drinking 30 minutes before taking your meals.
- It is recommended to take all the medicines according to the prescription of the doctor; nothing should be taken on your own. Taking any drug may initiate the formation of ulcers post-surgery.

- It is recommended to take approximately 60 grams of proteins every day post-surgery.
- Foods containing high fat or fiber content after the surgery are also prevented as the stomach needs to work too much to digest such substances that may produce stress in the body of the individual.
- It is also recommended to stop eating before satiety is achieved post-surgery.

You should not compel yourself to eat. It is ordinary during the underlying post-operation time to have almost no hunger. From the outset, it is likely for you to take in far less food than you may need, yet for the time being, it does not present a major issue. It is essential to keep yourself hydrated utilizing low to no calorie fluids and start utilizing food to show yourself new propensities that will assist you in adopting new habits and advance consistent weight reduction.

3.2 Creating a Diet that Works to Reduce Weight after Surgery

Formulating a diet plan that will work in reducing your weight after gastric bariatric surgery is not at all difficult if you follow the simple guidelines of what to eat and what to avoid after the surgery. There are some food materials that can be very tough to consume after the surgery though they are not avoided completely. Following are the guidelines that need to be followed for a diet that will help you reduce weight gradually without compromising your body needs for nutrients:

- Take proper meals containing all the food groups.
- Try to increase the intake of proteins in your diet as the body needs to strengthen after the surgery.
- Avoiding any sugar added foods is recommended.

- Try to avoid using straws while consuming your beverages as it adds air into the stomach, which causes discomfort and irritation later on.
- Drink extra water, but 30 minutes after your meal is over, eating between meals is highly prohibited.
- Try avoiding foods high in fiber, fats, or carbohydrates.
- Your daily caloric intake should not exceed the limit of 1000 calories.
- In the beginning, try to take in 300-400 calories, so your body does not have to do kind of excessive work.
- Two liters of fluid is recommended after the surgery. You can meet this target if you drink eight cups of water for the whole day.
- After the surgery, your body becomes highly sensitive to alcohol and is absorbed far more quickly than before, so alcoholic beverages are prohibited after the surgery.
- Try eating small portions of meat.
- It is recommended to chew slowly after the surgery.
- Snacking should be completely avoided after surgery for better weight loss results.
- It is also recommended to eat mindfully, i.e., eating while being occupied due to any work or the television is prohibited. Taking a break of one minute after each bite is encouraged by health care providers.
- Coconuts should be avoided completely; Milk products used should be low in lactose.
- Fruits and vegetables should be peeled before eating.
- Avoid using the white membranes, which are actually the fibers in citrus fruits such as oranges, grape fruits, and lemons.
- Tough meat is very difficult to chew, so instead, try to use tender meat and its products after surgery.
- Try to take toasted bread after surgery.
- Try to avoid caffeine, so tea and coffee are prohibited after gastric bariatric surgery.

- Fruit juices should be diluted into 50:50 ratios and then taken.

Following the above guidelines, you can quickly lose weight post-surgery and can lead a very healthy life ahead.

3.3 Therapeutic Diet- 30 Days Meal Plan

In this section, you will get a 30-day diet plan that you can follow to reduce further diet after the gastric bariatric surgery.

Day 1:
Breakfast: High Protein Smoothie   195 kcalories
Lunch: Chicken Broth   186 kcalories
Snack: Vanilla Probiotic Smoothie   183 kcalories
Dinner: Vegetable Broth 142 kcalories
Total Calories   706 kcalories

Day 2:
Breakfast: Mango and Pineapple Smoothie   197 kcalories
Lunch: White bean and Bone Broth   196 kcalories
Snack: Mango Smoothie 183 kcalories
Dinner: Tomato Soup   109 kcalories
Total Calories   685 kcalories

Day 3:
Breakfast: Blueberry Protein Smoothie   191 kcalories
Lunch: Kale and Chicken Broth Soup   212 kcalories
Snack: Tomato Smoothie123 kcalories
Dinner: Turkey Soup   190 kcalories
Total Calories   716 kcalories

Day 4:

Breakfast: Greek Yoghurt and Berry Smoothie   155 kcalories
Lunch: Pear and Butternut Soup   186 kcalories
Snack: Peach and Mango Smoothie   183 kcalories
Dinner: Parsnip Soup   220 kcalories
Total Calories   744 kcalories

Day 5:
Breakfast: Red Berry Smoothie   125 kcalories
Lunch: Mexican Taco Soup   204 kcalories
Snack: Strawberry and Banana smoothie   183 kcalories
Dinner: Chicken Broth   186 kcalories
Total Calories   698 kcalories

Day 6:
Breakfast: Tomato Smoothie   123 kcalories
Lunch: Vegetable Broth   142 kcalories
Snack: Green Juice   143 kcalories
Dinner: Creamy Chicken Soup   216 kcalories
Total Calories   624 kcalories

Day 7:
Breakfast: Black current and kale smoothie   186 kcalories
Lunch: White bean and Bone Broth   196 kcalories
Snack: Red Berry Smoothie   125 kcalories
Dinner: Vegetable Broth 142 kcalories
Total Calories   649 kcalories

Day 8:
Breakfast: Melon and Grape Juice   125 kcalories
Lunch: Turkey Soup   190 kcalories
Snack: Greek Yoghurt and Berry Smoothie   155 kcalories
Dinner: Tomato Soup   109 kcalories
Total Calories   579 kcalories

Day 9:

Breakfast: Blueberry juice   105 kcalories
Lunch: Kale and Chicken Broth Soup   212 kcalories
Snack: Blueberry Protein Smoothie   191 kcalories
Dinner: Broccoli and Potato Soup   179 kcalories
Total Calories   687 kcalories

Day 10:
Breakfast: Strawberry and Banana smoothie   183 kcalories
Lunch: Parsnip Soup   220 kcalories
Snack: Melon and Grape Juice   125 kcalories
Dinner: Vegetable Broth 142 kcalories
Total Calories   670 kcalories

Day 11:
Breakfast: Mango and Pineapple Smoothie   197 kcalories
Lunch: White bean and Bone Broth   196 kcalories
Snack: Vanilla Probiotic Smoothie   183 kcalories
Dinner: Vegetable Broth 142 kcalories
Total Calories718 kcalories

Day 12:
Breakfast: High Protein Smoothie   195 kcalories
Lunch: Chicken Broth   186 kcalories
Snack: Greek Yoghurt and Berry Smoothie   155 kcalories
Dinner: Tomato Soup   109 kcalories
Total Calories 645 kcalories

Day 13:
Breakfast: Red Berry Smoothie   125 kcalories
Lunch: Mexican Taco Soup   204 kcalories
Snack: Melon and Grape Juice   125 kcalories
Dinner: Vegetable Broth 142 kcalories
Total Calories596 kcalories

Day 14:
Breakfast: Black current and kale smoothie   186 kcalories
Lunch: White bean and Bone Broth   196 kcalories
Snack: Green Juice   143 kcalories
Dinner: Creamy Chicken Soup   216 kcalories
Total Calories741 kcalories

Day 15:
Breakfast: High Protein Smoothie   195 kcalories
Lunch: Chicken Broth   186 kcalories
Snack: Blueberry Protein Smoothie   191 kcalories
Dinner: Broccoli and Potato Soup   179 kcalories
Total Calories   761 kcalories

Day 16:
Breakfast: High Protein Smoothie   195 kcalories
Lunch: Mexican Taco Soup   204 kcalories
Snack: Strawberry and Banana smoothie   183 kcalories
Dinner: Chicken Broth   186 kcalories
Total Calories   678 kcalories

Day 17:
Breakfast: Melon and Grape Juice   125 kcalories
Lunch: White bean and Bone Broth 196 kcalories
Snack: Vanilla Probiotic Smoothie   183 kcalories
Dinner: Vegetable Broth142 kcalories
Total Calories   646 kcalories

Day 18:
Breakfast: High Protein Smoothie   195 kcalories
Lunch: Kale and Chicken Broth Soup   212 kcalories
Snack: Blueberry Protein Smoothie   191 kcalories
Dinner: Creamy Chicken Soup   216 kcalories
Total Calories   814 kcalories

Day 19:
Breakfast: Melon and Grape Juice   125 kcalories
Lunch: Chicken Broth   186 kcalories
Snack: Blueberry Protein Smoothie   191 kcalories
Dinner: Tomato Soup   109 kcalories
Total Calories   611 kcalories

Day 20:
Breakfast: Mango and Pineapple Smoothie   197 kcalories
Lunch: White bean and Bone Broth   196 kcalories
Snack: Green Juice   143 kcalories
Dinner: Kale and Chicken Broth Soup   212 kcalories
Total Calories   748 kcalories

Day 21:
Breakfast: High Protein Smoothie   195 kcalories
Lunch: Kale and Chicken Broth Soup212 kcalories
Snack: Blueberry Protein Smoothie   191 kcalories
Dinner: Chicken Broth   186 kcalories
Total Calories   784 kcalories

Day 22:
Breakfast: Vanilla Probiotic Smoothie   183 kcalories
Lunch: Vegetable Broth   142 kcalories
Snack: Tomato Smoothie 123 kcalories
Dinner: Turkey Soup   190 kcalories
Total Calories   638 kcalories

Day 23:
Breakfast: Blueberry   Protein   Smoothie   191 kcalories
Lunch: Creamy Chicken Soup   216 kcalories
Snack: Green Smoothie   183 kcalories
Dinner: Chicken Broth   186 kcalories
Total Calories   776 kcalories

Day 24:
Breakfast: Black current and kale smoothie   186 kcalories
Lunch: White bean and Bone Broth   196 kcalories
Snack: Red Berry Smoothie   125 kcalories
Dinner: Tomato Soup   109 kcalories
Total Calories   616 kcalories

Day 25:
Breakfast: Vanilla Probiotic Smoothie   183 kcalories
Lunch: Vegetable Broth142 kcalories
Snack: Peach and Mango Smoothie 183 kcalories
Dinner: Parsnip Soup   220 kcalories
Total Calories   728 kcalories

Day 26:
Breakfast: Melon and Grape Juice   125 kcalories
Lunch: Kale and Chicken Broth Soup   212 kcalories
Snack: Blueberry Protein Smoothie 191 kcalories
Dinner: Turkey Soup   190 kcalories
Total Calories   718 kcalories

Day 27:
Breakfast: Black current and kale smoothie   186 kcalories
Lunch: Pear and Butternut Soup   186 kcalories
Snack: Peach and Mango Smoothie 183 kcalories
Dinner: Chicken Broth 186 kcalories
Total Calories   741 kcalories

Day 28:
Breakfast: Vanilla Probiotic Smoothie   183 kcalories
Lunch: Parsnip Soup   220 kcalories
Snack: Melon and Grape Juice   125 kcalories
Dinner: Tomato Soup   109 kcalories
Total Calories   718 kcalories

Day 29:
Breakfast: Black current and kale smoothie   186 kcalories
Lunch: Vegetable Broth142 kcalories
Snack: Tomato Smoothie   123 kcalories
Dinner: Turkey Soup   190 kcalories
Total Calories   641 kcalories

Day 30:
Breakfast: Mango and Pineapple Smoothie   197 kcalories
Lunch: White bean and Bone Broth196 kcalories
Snack: Green Juice   143 kcalories
Dinner: Creamy Chicken Soup   216 kcalories
Total Calories   752 kcalories

The above 30-day therapeutic diet plan can be changed according to your choices and preferences by using the 100 different recipes below. Keep in mind the first 30- 40 days liquid diet is preferred to keep our stomach from working too much.

Chapter 4: 100 Different Recipes to Follow Post-Surgery

The time period post-surgery can be a very irritating one if your diet is not proper or as needed for the current condition. The gastric bariatric sleeve surgery can be very effective if the diet followed after the surgery is healthy, and according to the body's current needs. In this chapter, you will learn various healthy and easy to make recipes that you can make at home and feel healthy as well as reduce weight as you have always wanted.

4.1 Different Broth Recipes

Broths and soups are very healthy for the body and especially the stomach once it undergoes any surgery. This section contains fifteen different recipes that you can easily make by following the instructions in each recipe.

1) Chicken Broth

Preparation time: 15 minutes
Cooking time: 2 hours and 30 minutes
Serving: 4
Ingredients:

- Onion, diced, two medium-sized
- Carrots, diced, two medium-sized
- Celery, cut into chunks
- Dried thyme, one tsp.
- Rosemary dried, one tsp.
- Chicken with bone, two pounds
- Salt, according to your taste
- Water, two cups

Instructions:

1. Add all the above mentioned ingredients into a deep pan and bring it to boiling temperature.
2. Foam will form on the top layer, discard the foam, and cover the pan for about 2 hours 30 minutes.
3. Simmer the mixture for the above mentioned time on low heat.
4. Now discard the solids and then add salt into your soup.
5. Your soup is ready to be served.
6. You can enjoy it hot or at room temperature as you wish.

2) Creamy Chicken Soup

Preparation time: 15 minutes
Cooking time: 30 minutes
Serving: 1
Ingredients:
- Olive oil, one tbsp.
- Fresh chicken breast, cooked, one large
- Tomatoes, diced, two
- Carrots, diced, one
- Onion, diced, one
- Mushrooms, diced, two
- Chicken broth, two cups.
- Low fat sour cream, ½ cup
- Garlic powder, one tsp.
- Parsley, dried, one tsp.
- Sage, dried, one tsp.
- Rosemary, dried, one tsp.
- Thyme, dried, one tsp.
- Fennel, powdered form, one tsp.

Instructions:
1. Sautee the carrots and onions till they turn soft.
2. Add all the ingredients to the chicken broth and let it simmer for 15-20 minutes.
3. Add the sour cream and let it simmer for 5-10 minutes more.
4. Your soup is ready to be served.

3) White Bean and Bone Broth

Preparation time: 10 minutes
Cooking time: 40 minutes
Serving: 4
Ingredients:

- Extra virgin olive oil, one tbsp.
- Zucchini, small sized, one
- Carrot, diced, one
- Onion, diced, one medium sized
- Tomatoes, chopped, four medium sized
- Cloves of garlic, 3-4
- Spinach, one head
- Cannellini beans, one cup
- Chicken bone broth, two cups
- Cayenne pepper, one pinch
- Thyme, one tsp.
- Parsley, ¼ cup, chopped
- Basil, ¼ cup, chopped
- Beef gelation mixed with water, two tbsp.
- Parmesan cheese, according to your need
- Salt, for flavor

Instructions:

1. Add the oil in a pan and then add onion, when they turn soft and translucent add the garlic cloves and mix for a few minutes, now add all the spices along with the carrots into the pan and cook for one minute.
2. Add the zucchini and tomatoes and cook for one minute.
3. Add in the beans and the bone broth.
4. In the end, add the cheese, basil, parsley, and salt to taste and boil for one minute.
5. Your soup is ready to be served.

4) Kale and Chicken Broth Soup

Preparation time: 10 minutes
Cooking time: 1 hour and 30 minutes
Serving: 4
Ingredients:

- Onion, diced, two large
- Cabbage sliced, three cups
- Kale leaves, four, cut into large sizes
- Extra virgin olive oil, three tbsp.
- Chicken broth, two cups
- Shredded Chicken, two pounds
- Celery, two cups
- Parsley, dried, one tsp.
- Black pepper, one tsp.
- Oregano, dried, one tsp.
- Lemon juice, one tbsp.
- Garlic cloves, four

Instructions:

1. Take a deep pot or pan and add olive oil along with onions and carrots into it.
2. When they start to get, soft add the cabbage into it and cook for one minute.
3. Add the shredded chicken, chicken broth, and spices into it and make it into a soup.
4. Now add the kale, zucchini, and celery along with the lemon juice.
5. Simmer it for one hour on slow heat.
6. Your soup is ready to be served.
7. You can enjoy it either hot or at room temperature.

5) Vegetable Soup

Preparation time: 10 minutes
Cooking time: 18 minutes
Serving: 4
Ingredients:

- Carrots, diced, one cup
- Onions, diced, one cup
- Tomato puree, two tbsp.
- Cabbage chopped, four cups
- Green beans, one cup
- Garlic, minced, two cloves
- Bell peppers, two, chopped
- Beef broth, four cups
- Zucchini, one cup
- Broccoli, one cup
- Bay leaves, two
- Thyme, half tsp.
- Basil, half tsp.
- Salt to taste
- Pepper to taste

Instructions:

1. Take a pot and add the onions and carrots in oil till they turn soft.
2. Add in the carrots, green beans and cook them for five minutes.
3. Now add the rest of the stuff and simmer for 15-20 minutes till you see a mixture is formed.
4. Discard the bay leaves from your soup.
5. Your soup is ready to be served.

6) Mushroom and Kidney Beans Chicken Broth Soup

Preparation time: 20 minutes
Cooking time: 2 hours 30 minutes
Serving: 4-6
Ingredients:

- Carrots, diced, two cup
- Onions, diced, one small sized
- Tomato puree, two cups
- Mushroom chopped, one cup
- Kidney beans, one cup
- Garlic, minced, two cloves
- Cabbage, one, chopped
- Chicken broth, four cups
- Zucchini, one cup
- Italian seasoning, one tsp.
- Salt to taste

Instructions:

1. Add the mushrooms, carrots, onion, and oil in a pan and mix till they are soft.
2. Add the garlic and cook for a few minutes.
3. Now add the rest of the ingredients and let it simmer on low heat for approximately two hours.
4. Your soup is ready to be served.

7) Parsnip Soup

Preparation time: 20 minutes
Cooking time: 30 minutes
Serving: 4-6
Ingredients:

- Parsnip, 400 grams
- Vegetable stock cubes, two
- Semi Skimmed milk, 100 ml
- Boiling water, 400 ml
- Onion, diced, one large sized
- Salt and pepper to taste

Instructions:

1. Add onions in a pot with a little oil and cook till translucent.
2. Now add the water and vegetable stock cubes into the pot.
3. Add the parsnips into the pot and let it simmer for 20-25 minutes.
4. After this, blend all the ingredients with the help of a hand blender.
5. Add the milk and salt, pepper into the mixture, and your soup is ready to be served.

8) Pear and Butternut Soup

Preparation time: 20 minutes
Cooking time: 1 hour 20 minutes
Serving: 6-8
Ingredients:

- Extra virgin Olive oil, two tbsp.
- Pear, two small sized
- Sliced onion, one medium sized
- Butternut squash, one large
- Chicken broth, one cup
- Nonfat milk, one cup
- Thyme, three springs

Instructions:

1. Roast all the ingredients except the chicken broth and milk in a pre-heated oven for approximately 50-60 minutes.
2. Now remove the skin from all the ingredients and add it into a food processor to blend properly.
3. Add the blend into a pot with the chicken broth and let it boil for ten minutes.
4. Add the milk into the mixture and boil for 5-6 minutes.
5. Your soup is ready to be served.

9) Potato Soup

Preparation time: 10 minutes
Cooking time: 1 hour 5 minutes
Serving: 4
Ingredients:
- Extra virgin Olive oil, two tbsp.
- Potato, four small sized
- Sliced onion, one medium size
- Chicken broth, one cup
- Thyme, three springs

Instructions:

1. Roast all the ingredients except the chicken broth in a pre-heated oven for approximately 50-60 minutes.
2. Now remove the skin from all the ingredients and add it into a food processor to blend properly.
3. Add the blend into a pot with the chicken broth and let it boil for ten minutes.
4. Your soup is ready to be served.

10) Tomato Soup

Preparation time: 10 minutes
Cooking time: 1 hour 10 minutes
Serving: 4
Ingredients:
- Extra virgin Olive oil, two tbsp.
- Tomato, four large sized
- Sliced onion, one medium size
- Chicken broth, one cup
- Thyme, three springs

Instructions:
1. Roast all the ingredients except the chicken broth in a pre-heated oven for approximately 50-60 minutes.
2. Now remove the skin from all the ingredients and add it into a food processor to blend properly.
3. Add the blend into a pot with the chicken broth and let it boil for ten minutes.
4. Your soup is ready to be served.

11) Chicken and Potato Soup

Preparation time: 10 minutes
Cooking time: 1 hour 10 minutes
Serving: 4
Ingredients:
- Extra virgin Olive oil, two tbsp.
- Potato, four small sized
- Chicken Breast, two pounds
- Sliced onion, one medium size
- Chicken broth, one cup
- Thyme, three springs

Instructions:
1. Boil all the ingredients except the chicken broth on stove for approximately 50-60 minutes.
2. Now blend all of it by using a food processor.
3. Add the blend into a pot with the chicken broth and let it boil for ten minutes.
4. Your soup is ready to be served.

12) Broccoli and Potato Soup

Preparation time: 10 minutes
Cooking time: 1 hour 10 minutes
Serving: 3
Ingredients:
- Extra virgin Olive oil, two tbsp.
- Potato, four small sized
- Broccoli, one cup
- Sliced onion, one medium size
- Chicken broth, one cup
- Thyme, three springs

Instructions:
1. Roast all the ingredients except the chicken broth in a pre-heated oven for approximately 50-60 minutes.
2. Now blend all of it by using a food processor.
3. Add the blend into a pot with the chicken broth and let it boil for ten minutes.
4. Your soup is ready to be served.

13) Onion and Bean Soup

Preparation time: 10 minutes
Cooking time: 1 hour 10 minutes
Serving: 3
Ingredients:

- Extra virgin Olive oil, two tbsp.
- Onion, four small sized
- Kidney Beans, one cup
- Black Beans, one cup
- Chicken broth, one cup
- Thyme, three springs
- Salt to taste
- Pepper to taste

Instructions:

1. Boil the beans onion and thyme except for the chicken broth in a pre-heated oven for approximately 50-60 minutes.
2. Now blend all of it by using a food processor.
3. Add the blend into a pot with the chicken broth and let it boil for ten minutes.
4. Add the spices, i.e., salt and pepper.
5. Your soup is ready to be served.

14) Turkey Soup

Preparation time: 20 minutes
Cooking time: 60 minutes
Serving: 3
Ingredients:

- Extra virgin Olive oil, two tbsp.
- Onion, four small sized
- Mixed vegetables, one cup
- Mushrooms, half cup
- Tukey meat, two pounds
- Turkey broth, four cup
- Thyme, three springs
- Salt to taste
- Pepper to taste

Instructions:

1. Boil all the ingredients except the turkey broth on the stove for approximately 50 minutes.
2. Now blend all of it by using a food processor.
3. Add the blend into a pot with the turkey broth and let it boil for ten minutes.
4. Add the spices, i.e., salt and pepper.
5. Your soup is ready to be served.

15) Mexican Taco Soup

Preparation time: 10 minutes
Cooking time: 30 minutes
Serving: 3
Ingredients:
- Extra virgin Olive oil, two tbsp.
- Onion, four small sized
- Mixed vegetables, one cup
- Mushrooms, half cup
- Tukey meat, two pounds
- Chicken broth, four cup
- Tomatoes, two medium sized
- Garlic cloves, minced, two
- Taco seasoning, two tsp.
- Lemon juice, two tbsp.

Instructions:
1. Boil all the ingredients except the chicken broth on the stove for approximately 20 minutes.
2. Now blend all of it by using a food processor.
3. Add the blend into a pot with the chicken broth and let it boil for ten minutes.
4. Add the taco seasoning and lemon juice.
5. Your soup is ready to be served.

The soup recipes mentioned above are extremely delicious and very easy to make on your own.

4.2   Recipes for Smoothies

Following are some easy to make, healthy and delicious smoothie recipes that you can follow post bariatric surgery:

1) Mango and Pineapple Smoothie

Preparation time: 5 minutes
Serving: 1
Ingredients:
- Frozen mango chunks, ½ cup
- Frozen Pineapple chunks, ½ cup
- Vanilla ice cream, one scoop
- Low fat milk, one cup

Instructions:
1. Add all the ingredients in a blender and blend appropriately for three to four minutes.
2. Now pour into a cup and enjoy.
3. You can store this smoothie by freezing it.
4. Prior to using it later, you can re-blend the smoothie.

2) Banana and Chocolate Smoothie

Preparation time: 5 minutes

Serving: 1

Ingredients:

- Frozen banana chunks, ½ cup
- Frozen chocolate chunks, ½ cup
- Peanut Butter ice cream, one scoop
- Low fat milk, one cup

Instructions:

1. Add all the ingredients in a blender and blend appropriately for three to four minutes.
2. Now pour into a cup and enjoy.
3. You can store this smoothie by freezing it.
4. Prior to using it later, you can re-blend the smoothie.

3) Superfood Smoothie

Preparation time: 5 minutes
Serving: 1
Ingredients:
- Frozen kiwi chunks, ½ cup
- Fresh spinach, ½ cup
- Cucumber chunks, ¼ cup
- Chia seeds, one tsp.
- Low fat almond milk, one cup
- Vanilla protein powder, ½ cup

Instructions:
1. Add all the ingredients in a blender and blend appropriately for three to four minutes.
2. Now pour into a cup and enjoy.
3. You can store this smoothie by freezing it.
4. Prior to using it later, you can re-blend the smoothie.

4) Strawberry and Banana Smoothie

Preparation time: 5 minutes
Serving: 1
Ingredients:
- Frozen strawberry chunks, ½ cup
- Frozen banana chunks, ½ cup
- Peanut Butter ice cream, one scoop
- Low fat almond milk, one cup
- Vanilla protein powder, ½ cup

Instructions:
1. Add all the ingredients in a blender and blend appropriately for three to four minutes.
2. Now pour into a cup and enjoy.
3. You can store this smoothie by freezing it.
4. Prior to using it later, you can re-blend the smoothie.

5) Greek Yoghurt and Berry Smoothie

Preparation time: 5 minutes

Serving: 1

Ingredients:

- Frozen berries chunks, ½ cup
- Frozen Greek yoghurt, ½ cup
- Peanut Butter ice cream, one scoop
- Low fat almond milk, one cup
- Vanilla protein powder, ½ cup

Instructions:

1. Add all the ingredients in a blender and blend appropriately for three to four minutes.
2. Now pour into a cup and enjoy.
3. You can store this smoothie by freezing it.
4. Prior to using it later, you can re-blend the smoothie.

6) Pumpkin Spice Smoothie

Preparation time: 5 minutes

Serving: 1

Ingredients:

- Frozen pumpkin puree, ½ cup
- Cinnamon powder, ¼ tsp.
- Ground ginger powder, ¼ tsp.
- Ground cloves powder, ¼ tsp.
- Decaffeinated Coffee, ¾ cup
- Vanilla protein powder, 1/4cup
- Low fat milk, one cup

Instructions:

1. Add all the ingredients in a blender and blend appropriately for three to four minutes.
2. Now pour into a cup and enjoy.
3. You can store this smoothie by freezing it.
4. Prior to using it later, you can re-blend the smoothie.

7) Double Chocolate Smoothie

Preparation time: 5 minutes

Serving: 1

Ingredients:

- Frozen Greek Yoghurt, ½ cup
- Unsweetened Cocoa powder, ¼ tsp.
- Banana chunks, ¼ tsp.
- Chocolate protein powder, 1/4cup
- Low fat milk, one cup

Instructions:

1. Add all the ingredients in a blender and blend appropriately for three to four minutes.
2. Now pour into a cup and enjoy.
3. You can store this smoothie by freezing it.
4. Prior to using it later, you can re-blend the smoothie.

8) Probiotic Smoothie

Preparation time: 5 minutes

Serving: 1

Ingredients:

- Frozen Greek Yoghurt, ½ cup
- Plain Kefir, ½ cup
- Vanilla protein powder, ¼ cup
- Low fat milk, one cup

Instructions:

1. Add all the ingredients in a blender and blend appropriately for three to four minutes.
2. Now pour into a cup and enjoy.
3. You can store this smoothie by freezing it.
4. Prior to using it later, you can re-blend the smoothie.

9) Peanut Butter and Protein Smoothie

Preparation time: 5 minutes

Serving: 1

Ingredients:

- Frozen Greek Yoghurt, ½ cup
- Nonfat Ricotta Cheese, ½ cup
- Peanut Butter powder, ¼ cup
- Low fat milk, one cup
- Chocolate Protein powder, ¼ cup

Instructions:

1. Add all the ingredients in a blender and blend appropriately for three to four minutes.
2. Now pour into a cup and enjoy.
3. You can store this smoothie by freezing it.
4. Prior to using it later, you can re-blend the smoothie.

10) Apple Pie Smoothie

Preparation time: 5 minutes

Serving: 1

Ingredients:

- Frozen apple chunks, peeled, ½ cup
- Vanilla extract, one tsp.
- Cinnamon powder, ¼ tsp.
- Nutmeg powder, ¼ tsp.
- Low fat milk, one cup

Instructions:

1. Add all the ingredients in a blender and blend appropriately for three to four minutes.
2. Now pour into a cup and enjoy.
3. You can store this smoothie by freezing it.
4. Prior to using it later, you can re-blend the smoothie.

11) Red Berries Smoothie

Preparation time: 5 minutes

Serving: 1

Ingredients:

- Frozen red berries chunks, ½ cup
- Vanilla protein powder, ½ cup
- Low fat milk, one cup

Instructions:

1. Add all the ingredients in a blender and blend appropriately for three to four minutes.
2. Now pour into a cup and enjoy.
3. You can store this smoothie by freezing it.
4. Prior to using it later, you can re-blend the smoothie.

12) Peach and Mango Smoothie

Preparation time: 5 minutes

Serving: 1

Ingredients:

- Frozen mango chunks, ½ cup
- Vanilla protein powder, ½ cup
- Frozen Peach chunks, ½ cup
- Low fat milk, one cup

Instructions:

1. Add all the ingredients in a blender and blend appropriately for three to four minutes.
2. Now pour into a cup and enjoy.
3. You can store this smoothie by freezing it.
4. Prior to using it later, you can re-blend the smoothie.

13) Blueberry Protein Smoothie

Preparation time: 5 minutes

Serving: 1

Ingredients:

- Frozen blueberries chunks, ½ cup
- Vanilla protein powder, ½ cup
- Low fat milk, one cup

Instructions:

1. Add all the ingredients in a blender and blend appropriately for three to four minutes.
2. Now pour into a cup and enjoy.
3. You can store this smoothie by freezing it.
4. Prior to using it later, you can re-blend the smoothie.

14) Pear and Banana Protein Smoothie

Preparation time: 5 minutes

Serving: 1

Ingredients:

- Frozen banana chunks, ½ cup
- Vanilla protein powder, ½ cup
- Low fat milk, one cup
- Frozen Pear chunks, ½ cup

Instructions:

1. Add all the ingredients in a blender and blend appropriately for three to four minutes.
2. Now pour into a cup and enjoy.
3. You can store this smoothie by freezing it.
4. Prior to using it later, you can re-blend the smoothie.

15) Tomato Smoothie

Preparation time: 5 minutes

Serving: 1

Ingredients:

- Lemon juice, two tbsp.
- Carrot juice, ½ cup
- Tomato juice, one cup
- Tomatoes peeled, ½ cup
- Celery Stalk chopped, one

Instructions:

1. Add all the ingredients in a blender and blend appropriately for three to four minutes.
2. Now pour into a cup and enjoy.
3. You can store this smoothie by freezing it.
4. Prior to using it later, you can re-blend the smoothie.

Follow the amazing smoothie recipes mentioned above and make your surroundings healthy and nutritious.

4.3 Recipes for Salads

This section contains all the healthy salad recipes that you have always wanted. So, let us indulge in the world of healthy eating.

1) Chicken Salad

Preparation time: 10 minutes
Serving: 1
Ingredients:
- Olive oil based mayonnaise, one tbsp.
- Lemon juice, one tbsp.
- Low fat Greek yoghurt, two tbsp.
- Salt to taste
- Pepper to taste
- Cooked chicken, cubes, ½ cup

Instructions:
1. Add the liquid based ingredients in a bowl and mix together to make a paste.
2. Now add the chicken cubes and combine to form a salad.
3. Add salt and pepper according to your taste.
4. Your salad is ready to be served.

2) Classic Tuna Salad

Preparation time: 10 minutes

Serving: 1

Ingredients:

- Olive oil based mayonnaise, one tbsp.
- Lemon juice, one tbsp.
- Low fat Greek yoghurt, two tbsp.
- Salt to taste
- Pepper to taste
- Cooked tuna, cubes, ½ cup
- Dijon mustard, one tbsp.
- Red onion, chopped, one tbsp.
- Finely chopped pickles, one tbsp.

Instructions:

1. Add the liquid based ingredients in a bowl and mix together to make a paste.
2. Now add the tuna cubes, chopped pickles, onion, and mix to form a salad.
3. Add salt and pepper according to your taste.
4. Your salad is ready to be served.

3) Tomato, Cucumber and Basil Salad

Preparation time: 10 minutes

Serving: 1

Ingredients:

- Olive oil based mayonnaise, one tbsp.
- Lemon juice, one tbsp.
- Red onion, chopped, one
- Low fat Greek yoghurt, two tbsp.
- Pepper to taste
- Cucumber, cubes, ½ cup
- Dijon mustard, one tbsp.
- Tomatoes, chopped, 1 cup
- Finely chopped basil, ½ cup

Instructions:

1. Add the liquid based ingredients in a bowl and mix together to make a paste.
2. Now add the tomato, cucumber, chopped basil, onion, and mix to form a salad.
3. Add pepper according to your taste.
4. Your salad is ready to be served.

4) Roasted Vegetable Quinoa and Chickpea Salad

Preparation time: 10 minutes
Cooking time: 35 minutes
Serving: 1
Ingredients:

- Vegetable broth, one cup
- Quinoa, ½ cup
- Summer squash, chopped, one
- Cooked chickpeas, one cup
- Dried oregano, one tsp.
- Zucchini, diced, ½ cup
- Dried basil, one tbsp.
- Eggplants, diced, ½ cup
- Finely chopped tomatoes, ½ cup

Instructions:

1. Bake all the vegetables in an oven for about 30 minutes.
2. Add the quinoa and broth in a pan and let it boil when the vegetables are being roasted.
3. Boil it until the liquid is absorbed.
4. Now mix all the ingredients together, adding the spices and roasted vegetables and chickpeas.
5. Your salad is ready to be served.

5) Shrimp Salad

Preparation time: 10 minutes
Cooking time: 5 minutes
Serving: 1
Ingredients:

- Half lemon
- Shrimp, one pound
- Cucumber, chopped, one
- Dried thyme, one tsp.
- Seafood sauce, ½ cup
- Dried basil, one tbsp.
- Lettuce, diced, ½ cup
- Low fat Greek yoghurt, three tbsp.
- Olive oil based mayonnaise, ½ cup
- Bay leaf, one

Instructions:

1. Fill a deep pan with water and add thyme, bay leaves, lemon juice, shrimp, and dried basil into the boiling water.
2. Drain the shrimp once cooked and let it cool down.
3. In a large bowl, mix the Greek yoghurt, mayonnaise, and seafood sauce.
4. Now add the cucumber and lettuce.
5. Add the cooled shrimps on top of the salad.
6. Your salad is ready to be served.

6) Cucumber, Avocado, Black bean, Corn and Tomato Salad

Preparation time: 10 minutes

Serving: 1

Ingredients:

- Olive oil based mayonnaise, one tbsp.
- Lemon juice, one tbsp.
- Corn, one cup
- Black beans, one cup
- Low fat Greek yoghurt, two tbsp.
- Pepper to taste
- Cucumber, cubes, ½ cup
- Dijon mustard, one tbsp.
- Tomatoes, chopped, 1 cup
- Finely chopped avocado, ½ cup

Instructions:

1. Add the liquid based ingredients in a bowl and mix together to make a paste.
2. Now add the tomato, cucumber, avocado, corn, black beans, and mix to form a salad.
3. Add pepper according to your taste.
4. Your salad is ready to be served.

7) Baby Arugula and Parmesan Salad

Preparation time: 10 minutes

Serving: 1

Ingredients:

- Olive oil based mayonnaise, one tbsp.
- Lemon juice, one tbsp.
- Baby Arugula, one cup
- Parmesan cheese, one cup
- Low fat Greek yoghurt, two tbsp.
- Pepper to taste

Instructions:

1. Add the liquid based ingredients in a bowl and mix together to make a paste.
2. Now add the baby arugula, parmesan cheese, and mix to form a salad.
3. Add pepper according to your taste.
4. Your salad is ready to be served.

8) Bacon and Avocado Salad

Preparation time: 10 minutes

Serving: 1

Ingredients:

- Olive oil based mayonnaise, one tbsp.
- Lemon juice, one tbsp.
- Cooked Bacon, cut into small pieces, one cup
- Avocado, diced, one cup
- Low fat Greek yoghurt, two tbsp.
- Pepper to taste

Instructions:

1. Add the liquid based ingredients in a bowl and mix together to make a paste.
2. Now add the bacon, avocado, and mix to form a salad.
3. Add pepper according to your taste.
4. Your salad is ready to be served.

9) Shrimp and Tomato Spinach Salad

Preparation time: 10 minutes

Cooking time: 5 minutes

Serving: 1

Ingredients:

- Half lemon
- Shrimp, one pound
- Tomato, chopped, one
- Dried thyme, one tsp.
- Seafood sauce, ½ cup
- Dried basil, one tbsp.
- Baby spinach, ½ cup
- Low fat Greek yoghurt, three tbsp.
- Olive oil based mayonnaise, ½ cup
- Bay leaf, one

Instructions:

1. Fill a deep pan with water and add bay leaves, lemon juice, shrimp, and dried basil into the boiling water.
2. Drain the shrimp once cooked and let it cool down.
3. In a large bowl, mix the Greek yoghurt, mayonnaise, and seafood sauce.
4. Now add the tomatoes and spinach.
5. Add the cooled shrimps on top of the salad.
6. Your salad is ready to be served.

10) Chicken, Potato and Green Bean Salad

Preparation time: 10 minutes

Serving: 1

Ingredients:

- Olive oil based mayonnaise, one tbsp.
- Lemon juice, one tbsp.
- Low fat Greek yoghurt, two tbsp.
- Salt to taste
- Pepper to taste
- Cooked chicken, cubes, ½ cup
- Dijon mustard, one tbsp.
- Red potato, cooked and chopped, one tbsp.
- Green beans, cooked, one cup

Instructions:

1. Add the liquid based ingredients in a bowl and mix together to make a paste.
2. Now add the chicken, beans, potatoes, and mix to form a salad.
3. Add pepper according to your taste.
4. Your salad is ready to be served.

11) Grilled Chicken and Wheat berry Salad

Preparation time: 10 minutes

Serving: 1

Ingredients:

- Olive oil based mayonnaise, one tbsp.
- Lemon juice, one tbsp.
- Low fat Greek yoghurt, two tbsp.
- Salt to taste
- Pepper to taste
- Grilled chicken, two breasts
- Dijon mustard, one tbsp.
- Cooked wheat berries, one cup

Instructions:

1. Add the liquid based ingredients in a bowl and mix together to make a paste.
2. Now add the wheat berries and mix to form a salad.
3. Place the grilled chicken pieces on top of the salad.
4. Add pepper according to your taste.
5. Your salad is ready to be served.

12) Balsamic Watermelon and Chicken Salad

Preparation time: 10 minutes

Serving: 1

Ingredients:

- Olive oil, one tbsp.
- Lemon juice, one tbsp.
- Baby Spinach, one cup
- All-purpose seasoning, one tsp.
- Pepper to taste
- Watermelon cubes
- Grilled chicken, two breasts
- Dijon mustard, one tbsp.
- Balsamic Vinegar, one tsp
- Crushed almonds, 5-6
- Blue cheese crumbles, three tbsp.

Instructions:

1. Add the liquid based ingredients in a bowl and mix together to make a paste.
2. Now add the watermelon, spinach, blue cheese, and mix to form a salad.
3. Place the grilled chicken pieces on top of the salad.
4. Add pepper according to your taste.
5. Your salad is ready to be served.

13) Strawberry and Spinach Salad

Preparation time: 10 minutes

Serving: 1

Ingredients:

- Olive oil, one tbsp.
- Lemon juice, one tbsp.
- Baby Spinach, one cup
- All-purpose seasoning, one tsp.
- Pepper to taste
- Strawberry cubes, one cup
- Dijon mustard, one tbsp.

Instructions:

1. Add the liquid based ingredients in a bowl and mix together to make a paste.
2. Now add the strawberry, spinach, and mix to form a salad.
3. Add pepper according to your taste.
4. Your salad is ready to be served.

14) Salmon, Blue Cheese, and Baby Spinach Salad

Preparation time: 10 minutes

Serving: 1

Ingredients:

- Olive oil, one tbsp.
- Lemon juice, one tbsp.
- Baby Spinach, one cup
- All-purpose seasoning, one tsp.
- Pepper to taste
- Grilled Salmon, two pounds
- Dijon mustard, one tbsp.
- Balsamic Vinegar, one tsp
- Crushed almonds, 5-6
- Blue cheese crumbles, three tbsp.

Instructions:

1. Add the liquid based ingredients in a bowl and mix together to make a paste.
2. Now add the blue cheese, spinach, and mix to form a salad.
3. Place the grilled salmon pieces on top of the salad.
4. Add pepper according to your taste.
5. Your salad is ready to be served.

15) Carrot and Pineapple Salad

Preparation time: 10 minutes

Serving: 1

Ingredients:

- Olive oil, one tbsp.
- Lemon juice, one tbsp.
- Carrot, diced, one cup
- All-purpose seasoning, one tsp.
- Pepper to taste
- Pineapple, diced, one cup
- Dijon mustard, one tbsp.
- Balsamic Vinegar, one tsp
- Crushed almonds, 5-6
- Blue cheese crumbles, three tbsp.

Instructions:

1. Add the liquid based ingredients in a bowl and mix together to make a paste.
2. Now add the blue cheese, carrots, pineapples, and mix to form a salad.
3. Add pepper according to your taste.
4. Your salad is ready to be served.

The above mentioned salad recipes are very healthy. They are easy to make on your own after going through the bariatric surgery. You can easily change your lifestyle by adopting the easy to make recipes. You can continue losing weight and feeling healthy as well as sound for a long period as your diet is directly linked to your mood.

4.4 Breakfast Recipes

This section contains all the healthy recipes that you can follow after a gastric bariatric surgery. You can make them at home by following the simple instructions and get a fresh as well as a healthy start to your day.

1) Cinnamon Oatmeal

Preparation time: 10 minutes
Cooking time: 7 hours
Serving: 7-8
Ingredients:

- Oats, two cups
- Water, eight cups
- Peanut butter powder, two tbsp.
- Nutmeg, ground form, one tsp.
- Cinnamon powder, one tsp.
- Low fat milk, one cup
- Pumpkin puree, ¼ cup
- Sliced mixed fruit, ½ cup
- Frozen or fresh berries, half cup
- Vanilla protein powder, two tbsp.
- Nonfat milk powder, two tbsp.

Instructions:

1. In a deep pan, add the water, oats, cinnamon, and nutmeg and let it cook over low heat for 7 hours approximately.
2. Now when cooked, add milk, peanut butter powder, pumpkin puree, vanilla protein powder, nonfat milk powder, and then cook it for 2-3 minutes.
3. Remove it in a bowl and then add the mixed fruit slices and berries on top and enjoy.
4. Your dish is ready to be served.

2) Vanilla and Cherry Baked Oatmeal

Preparation time: 10 minutes

Cooking time: 45 minutes

Serving: 6

Ingredients:

- Oats, one cups
- Water, eight cups
- Peanut butter powder, two tbsp.
- Nutmeg, ground form, one tsp.
- Flaxseed powder, one tbsp.
- Low fat milk, one cup
- Low fat Greek yoghurt, ½ cup
- Eggs, 3
- Fresh cherries one cup
- Baking powder, ¾ tsp.
- Vanilla extract, one tsp.
- Liquid stevia, one tsp.
- Apple, chopped, one

Instructions:

1. Mix the dry ingredients in a bowl and the wet ingredients in a separate bowl.
2. Preheat the oven at 375 degrees for twenty minutes.
3. Now mix the ingredients together and then add cherries.
4. Fold the mixture and add it into a non-stick pan.
5. Place the pan in the oven for 45 minutes until edges turn crispy and are adequately cooked.
6. Your dish is ready to be served.

3) Cheese Pancakes

Preparation time: 5 minutes
Cooking time: 5 minutes
Serving: 2
Ingredients:
- Low fat cottage cheese, one cup
- Eggs, 3
- Coconut oil, melted, one and a half tbsp.
- Whole wheat flour, half cup
- Non-stick spray for cooking

Instructions:
1. Mix the eggs in a bowl.
2. Add the wheat flour, coconut oil, and cheese and mix properly.
3. Now spray a non-stick pan.
4. Add some of the batter and cook on each side till the color turns light brown.
5. Your pancakes are ready to be served.

4) Pumpkin, Zucchini and Walnuts Muffins

Preparation time: 10 minutes

Cooking time: 25 minutes

Serving: 6

Ingredients:

- Oats, two cups
- Pumpkin puree, ½ cup
- Nutmeg, ground form, ¼ tsp.
- All spice, ground form, ¼ tsp.
- Flaxseed powder, one tbsp.
- Low fat milk, one cup
- Low fat Greek yoghurt, ½ cup
- Eggs, 4
- Shredded zucchini, one cup
- Baking powder, two tbsp.
- Vanilla extract, one tsp.
- Liquid stevia, one tsp.
- Baking soda, ½ tsp.
- Walnuts, chopped, half cup

Instructions:

1. Preheat the oven at 375 degrees for 20 minutes.
2. Mix the dry and wet ingredients separately first and then add the dry ingredients to the wet ingredients slowly folded the mixture.
3. Add the zucchini and walnuts into the bowl and fold.
4. Now use a muffins tray and line it with butter paper and some nonstick spray.
5. Add the mixture in each muffin holder and place it in the oven for 25 minutes.
6. Remove it from the oven once cooked.
7. Your muffins are ready to be served.

5) Scrambled Eggs with Tukey and Cheddar Cheese

Preparation time: 10 minutes

Cooking time: 10 minutes

Serving: 3

Ingredients:

- Garlic powder, ground form, ¼ tsp.
- Onion powder, ground form, ¼ tsp.
- Cheddar cheese, three oz.
- Low fat turkey, eight oz.
- Eggs, 6

Instructions:

1. Cook the turkey pieces for approximately 5-7 minutes until they turn light brown.
2. Now spray a pan with cooking oil and add the beaten eggs with garlic and onion powder into it.
3. Top it with turkey pieces and shredded cheddar cheese.
4. Cook it properly by mixing it.
5. Your eggs are ready to be served.

6) Eggs with Cauliflower

Preparation time: 10 minutes
Cooking time: 10 minutes
Serving: 3
Ingredients:

- Oil, one tsp.
- Deli ham, three oz.
- Cooked cauliflower pieces, eight oz.
- Eggs, 2

Instructions:

1. Cook the ham pieces for approximately 5-7 minutes until they turn light brown.
2. Now spray a pan with cooking oil and add the beaten eggs with cauliflower into it.
3. Cook it properly by flipping it.
4. Top it with ham pieces.
5. Your eggs are ready to be served.

7) Scrambled Egg Burrito:

Preparation time: 10 minutes

Cooking time: 10 minutes

Serving: 6

Ingredients:

- Extra virgin olive oil, one tsp.
- Cooked black beans, twelve oz.
- Eggs, 12
- Bell pepper, diced, one
- Low fat milk, ¼ cup
- Salsa, for serving
- Low wheat Tortillas, 6

Instructions:

1. Add olive oil in a pan with cooking oil and add the beaten eggs with beans, milk, and bell pepper into it.
2. Cook it properly by mixing it.
3. Top it with salsa.
4. Add everything into the low wheat tortillas and make a burrito.
5. Your dish is ready to be served.

8) Egg Casserole with Onions, Mushrooms, and Broccoli

Preparation time: 10 minutes
Cooking time: 40 minutes
Serving: 6
Ingredients:

- Onions, chopped, one cup
- Cooked mushrooms, twelve oz.
- Eggs, 12
- Broccoli, diced, one cup
- Low fat milk, ¼ cup
- Shredded cheese, one cup
- Dried oregano, ½ tsp.
- Dried thyme, ½ tsp.
- Dried basil. ½ tsp.
- Shredded chicken, one cup

Instructions:

1. Add the onions into a pan to be cooked until translucent. Add the broccoli and mushrooms and cook for a few minutes.
2. Preheat the oven at 375 degrees.
3. In a large bowl mix in the herbs, milk, and eggs.
4. Add the shredded cheese, chicken, and cooked vegetables into it.
5. Now add this mixture into a nonstick pan and bake it for 30-35 minutes.
6. Your dish is ready to be served.

9) Scrambled Eggs with Ricotta Cheese and Chives

Preparation time: 10 minutes

Cooking time: 10 minutes

Serving: 3

Ingredients:

- Extra virgin olive oil, one tsp.
- Eggs, 6
- Chives, half cup
- Ricotta cheese, half cup
- Low fat milk, ¼ cup

Instructions:

1. Add olive oil in a pan with cooking oil and add the beaten eggs with chives and milk into it
2. Cook it properly by mixing it.
3. Add the ricotta cheese.
4. Cook it for a few minutes and dish it out.
5. Your dish is ready to be served.

10) Spinach and Egg Scramble

Preparation time: 10 minutes

Cooking time: 10 minutes

Serving: 3

Ingredients:

- Extra virgin olive oil, one tsp.
- Eggs, 6
- Baby spinach, one cup
- Low fat milk, ¼ cup

Instructions:

1. Add olive oil in a pan with cooking oil and add the beaten eggs with milk into it
2. Cook it properly by mixing it.
3. Add spinach into it.
4. Cook it for a few minutes and dish it out.
5. Your dish is ready to be served.

11) Cottage Cheese Scrambled Eggs

Preparation time: 10 minutes

Cooking time: 10 minutes

Serving: 3

Ingredients:

- Extra virgin olive oil, one tsp.
- Eggs, 6
- Shredded cottage cheese, one cup
- Low fat milk, ¼ cup

Instructions:

1. Add olive oil in a pan with cooking oil and add the beaten eggs with milk into it
2. Cook it properly by mixing it.
3. Add cottage cheese into it.
4. Cook it for a few minutes and dish it out.
5. Your dish is ready to be served.

12) Eggs with Avocado

Preparation time: 10 minutes

Cooking time: 10 minutes

Serving: 3

Ingredients:

- Extra virgin olive oil, one tsp.
- Eggs, 6
- Avocado slices
- Low fat milk, ¼ cup

Instructions:

1. Add olive oil in a pan with cooking oil and add the beaten eggs with milk into it
2. Cook it properly by mixing it.
3. Cook it for a few minutes and dish it out.
4. Place the avocado slices on top.
5. Your dish is ready to be served.

13) Bacon and Eggs

Preparation time: 10 minutes
Cooking time: 5 minutes
Serving: 1
Ingredients:
- Extra virgin olive oil, one tsp.
- Eggs, 2
- Cooked bacon slices
- Salt to taste
- Pepper to taste

Instructions:
1. Add the oil in a pan and break the egg on top of it.
2. Cook it for two minutes and dish out.
3. Add salt and pepper according to your taste.
4. Served it with slices for cooked bacon.

14) Strawberry and Blueberry Oatmeal

Preparation time: 10 minutes

Cooking time: 7 hours

Serving: 7-8

Ingredients:

- Oats, two cups
- Water, eight cups
- Peanut butter powder, two tbsp.
- Nutmeg, ground form, one tsp.
- Cinnamon powder, one tsp.
- Low fat milk, one cup
- Pumpkin puree, ¼ cup
- Blueberries, ½ cup
- Strawberries, ½ cup
- Vanilla protein powder, two tbsp.
- Nonfat milk powder, two tbsp.

Instructions:

1. In a deep pan, add the water, oats, cinnamon, and nutmeg and let it cook over low heat for 7 hours approximately.
2. Now when cooked, add milk, peanut butter powder, pumpkin puree, vanilla protein powder, nonfat milk powder, and then cook it for 2-3 minutes.
3. Remove it in a bowl and then add the strawberries and blueberries on top and enjoy.
4. Your dish is ready to be served.

15) Blueberry Protein Pancakes

Preparation time: 5 minutes
Cooking time: 5 minutes
Serving: 2
Ingredients:

- Blueberries, one cup
- Eggs, 3
- Coconut oil, melted, one and a half tbsp.
- Whole wheat flour, half cup
- Vanilla protein powder, two tbsp.
- Non-stick spray for cooking

Instructions:

1. Mix the eggs in a bowl.
2. Add the wheat flour, vanilla protein powder, coconut oil, blueberries, and mix properly.
3. Now spray a non-stick pan.
4. Add some of the batter and cook on each side till the color turns light brown.
5. Your pancakes are ready to be served.

16) Apple Pie Oatmeal

Preparation time: 10 minutes
Cooking time: 7 hours
Serving: 7-8
Ingredients:

- Oats, two cups
- Water, eight cups
- Peanut butter powder, two tbsp.
- Nutmeg, ground form, one tsp.
- Cinnamon powder, one tsp.
- Low fat milk, one cup
- Pumpkin puree, ¼ cup
- Apple, ½ cup
- Vanilla protein powder, two tbsp.
- Nonfat milk powder, two tbsp.

Instructions:

1. In a deep pan, add the water, oats, cinnamon, and nutmeg and let it cook over low heat for 7 hours approximately.
2. Now when cooked, add milk, peanut butter powder, pumpkin puree, vanilla protein powder, nonfat milk powder, and then cook it for 2-3 minutes.
3. Remove it in a bowl and then add the diced apples on top and enjoy.
4. Your dish is ready to be served.

17) Baked Egg, Chicken and Cheese Casserole

Preparation time: 10 minutes
Cooking time: 40 minutes
Serving: 6
Ingredients:

- Eggs, 12
- Shredded cottage cheese, one cup
- Low fat milk, ¼ cup
- Shredded ricotta cheese, one cup
- Dried oregano, ½ tsp.
- Dried thyme, ½ tsp.
- Dried basil. ½ tsp.
- Shredded chicken, one cup

Instructions:

1. Preheat the oven at 375 degrees.
2. In a large bowl mix in the herbs, milk, and eggs.
3. Add the shredded cheese and chicken into it.
4. Now add this mixture into a nonstick pan and bake it for 30-35 minutes.
5. Your dish is ready to be served.

18) Protein French Toast

Preparation time: 10 minutes
Cooking time: 5 minutes
Serving: 4
Ingredients:

- Eggs, two
- Peanut butter powder, two tbsp.
- Nutmeg, ground form, one tsp.
- Low fat milk, one cup
- Vanilla protein powder, two tbsp.
- Nonfat milk powder, two tbsp.
- Fresh fruits, half cup
- Olive oil, two tbsp.
- Bran bread, four slices
- Maple syrup according to taste

Instructions:

1. In a bowl, mix the eggs, peanut butter powder, low fat milk, nutmeg powder, vanilla protein powder, nonfat milk powder together and mix well.
2. Now add the oil in a pan and heat.
3. Soak the bread in the mixture of eggs and fry in the pan till golden brown.
4. Place the fresh fruits and pour the maple syrup on the bread slices.
5. Your dish is ready to be served.

The breakfast recipes mentioned above are very healthy, easy to make. You can give your daily routine a fresh boost by following these delicious recipes.

4.5 Lunch Recipes

In this section, you will find amazing lunch recipes by the following the simple and easy instructions mentioned for each recipe.

1) Mexican Style Stuffed Summer Squash

Preparation time: 5 minutes
Cooking time: 33 minutes
Serving: 2
Ingredients:
- Refried black beans, ½ cup
- Cooked Quinoa, ½ cup
- Tomato, diced, one small sized
- Black olives, sliced, two tbsp.
- Scallions, chopped, two
- Shredded Colby jack cheese, one cup
- Non-stick spray

Instructions:
1. Preheat the oven at 400 Fahrenheit.
2. Place the summer squash in a baking dish by firstly removing the inside material. Gently poke it before baking. Bake for three to four minutes.
3. Mix the rest of the stuff together and place the stuffing in the summer squash.
4. Add the cheese on top and bake for 20 minutes.
5. When baked, dish out and add the chopped scallions on top.
6. Your meal is ready to be served.

2) Barley and Mushroom Risotto

Preparation time: 5 minutes
Cooking time: 55 minutes
Serving: 6
Ingredients:

- Garlic, minced, one tsp.
- Leaks, diced, two
- Extra virgin olive oil, one tbsp.
- Sliced mushrooms, four cups
- Fresh spinach leaves, three cups
- White wine, half cup
- Chicken broth, one cup
- Barley, half cup
- Thyme, two tsp.

Instructions:

1. In a large deep pan, add the olive oil and garlic. Cook it for a few seconds and add the leeks and mushrooms.
2. Add the barley and thyme and cook for a few minutes.
3. Add the wine and mix it properly.
4. Add the broth and let it simmer for 30 minutes on low heat.
5. Now add the spinach and mix till they are wilted.
6. Your dish is ready to be served.

3) Coconut and Tofu Curry

Preparation time: 15 minutes
Cooking time: 30 minutes
Serving: 6
Ingredients:
- Grated ginger, one tbsp.
- Minced garlic, one tbsp.
- Cinnamon, quarter tsp.
- Turmeric, half tsp.
- Curry powder, two tsp.
- Ground cumin, half tsp.
- Coconut oil, three tbsp.
- Extra firm tofu, 14 oz.
- Unsweetened coconut milk, two cups
- Tomato puree, one cup
- Carrots, diced, two
- Bok Choi, two stems
- Chicken broth, two cups
- Fresh cilantro, half cup

Instructions:
1. Cook the tofu cubes in the coconut oil for 3-4 minutes till a firm layer forms on the tofu cubes.
2. Add the rest of the ingredients by first removing the tofu from the pan.
3. Mix the coconut milk into it. Now add the tofu and bok choi into the mixture and cook it for few minutes.
4. Serve it with rice and garnish it with fresh cilantro.

4) Eggplant Rollatini

Preparation time: 15 minutes

Cooking time: 50 minutes

Serving: 6

Ingredients:

- Eggplant, one large
- Salt, one tbsp.
- Extra virgin olive oil, one tsp.
- Fresh spinach, 10 cups
- Mozzarella cheese, half cup
- Ricotta cheese, half cup
- Minced garlic, one tsp.
- Egg, one
- Marinara sauce, one cup
- Parmigianino Reggiano cheese, one cup

Instructions:

1. Add the salt on the eggplant by cutting it into half. Let it be for 10 minutes.
2. Now wash off the salt and place the eggplant in a preheated oven for 10 minutes.
3. In a large pan, add the olive oil, garlic, and spinach, cook it till wilted.
4. Now in a baking dish, add the marinara sauce, eggplant, and spinach one by one.
5. Top it with cheese, cover with an aluminum foil and bake for 30 minutes.
6. Remove the foil and bake it for an extra 10 minutes.
7. Your dish is ready to be served.

5) Eggplant, Chickpea, and Quinoa Curry

Preparation time: 15 minutes

Cooking time: 20 minutes

Serving: 6-8

Ingredients:

- Eggplant, one large, cut into chunks
- Summer squash, one large, cut into chunks
- Tomato, diced, three medium sized
- Ground cumin, one tbsp.
- Extra virgin olive oil, one tsp.
- Onion, chopped, one large sized
- Bell pepper, chopped, one large sized
- Vegetable broth, one cup
- Water, half cup
- Minced garlic, four tsp.
- Turmeric, one tsp.
- Cayenne pepper, half tsp.
- Smoked paprika, half tsp.
- Chickpeas, cooked, one cup
- Quinoa, cooked, half cup

Instructions:

1. Take a large pan, add the onions and garlic and cook.
2. Now, add the vegetables and tomatoes into it cook for few minutes.
3. Add the water, vegetable broth, chickpeas, and spices.
4. Simmer it on a low stove for about ten to fifteen minutes.
5. Serve them on top of the quinoa.
6. Your dish is ready to be served.

6) Cauliflower and Cheese Casserole

Preparation time: 10 minutes

Cooking time: 45 minutes

Serving: 6-8

Ingredients:

- Low fat Greek yoghurt, one cup
- Cauliflower, partially cooked, two cups, cut into chunks
- Dijon mustard, one tbsp.
- Garlic powder, one tbsp.
- Shredded aged cheddar cheese, one cup
- Shredded mozzarella cheese, half cup

Instructions:

1. Preheat the oven for about 400 Fahrenheit.
2. Mix the yoghurt, garlic powder, Dijon mustard, and cauliflower together and add it in a baking dish.
3. Top it with cheese and cover it with an aluminum foil. Now, bake it for 35 minutes.
4. Remove the foil and broil it for 10 minutes.
5. Your dish is ready to be served.

7) Basil and Garlic Grilled Chicken

Preparation time: 10 minutes
Cooking time: 25 minutes
Serving: 2
Ingredients:

- Low fat Greek yoghurt, one cup
- Chicken breast, two pounds
- Dijon mustard, one tbsp.
- Garlic powder, one tbsp.
- Dried basil, one tsp.
- Salt to taste
- Olive oil, two tbsp.

Instructions:

1. Take a large bowl and mix all the ingredients together.
2. Now add the olive oil on a grill and place the chicken pieces on it.
3. Cook on each side.
4. Cut into pieces and serve with grilled vegetables of your choice.
5. You can also serve it along with rice.

8) Black Bean and Butternut Squash Enchiladas

Preparation time: 15 minutes
Cooking time: 40 minutes
Serving: 2-4
Ingredients:
- Garlic, minced, one tsp.
- Butternut squash, diced, one
- Bell pepper, diced, one
- Jalapeno pepper, diced, one
- Low sodium taco seasoning, one tsp.
- Extra virgin olive oil, two tbsp.
- Onion, diced, one
- Black beans, cooked, two cups
- Enchilada sauce, one cup
- Black olives, sliced, half cup
- Tomatoes, diced, two medium sized
- Whole wheat tortilla, eight
- Scallions, chopped for garnishing
- Cheddar cheese, shredded, one cup

Instructions:
1. Preheat the oven at 400 Fahrenheit.
2. Now add the olive oil, garlic, and onions. Cook for a few minutes.
3. Add the vegetables and cook the mixture.
4. Now add the enchilada sauce in a baking dish and line the tortillas on it. Add the cooked mixture and cheddar cheese on it and bake for 30 minutes.
5. Your dish is ready to be served.
6. Add the scallions on top for garnishing.

9) Tuna Casserole

Preparation time: 10 minutes
Cooking time: 35 minutes
Serving: 6-8
Ingredients:
- Low fat Greek yoghurt, one cup
- Tuna, partially cooked, two cups, cut into chunks
- Dijon mustard, one tbsp.
- Garlic powder, one tbsp.
- Shredded aged cheddar cheese, one cup
- Shredded mozzarella cheese, half cup

Instructions:
1. Preheat the oven for about 400 Fahrenheit.
2. Mix the yoghurt, garlic powder, Dijon mustard and tuna together and add it in a baking dish.
3. Top it with cheese and cover it with an aluminum foil. Now, bake it for 35 minutes.
4. Remove the foil and broil it for 10 minutes.
5. Your dish is ready to be served.

10) Herb Roasted Salmon

Preparation time: 10 minutes
Cooking time: 25 minutes
Serving: 2
Ingredients:

- Low fat Greek yoghurt, one cup
- Salmon, two pounds
- Dijon mustard, one tbsp.
- Garlic powder, one tbsp.
- Dried basil, one tsp.
- Thyme, two leaves
- Oregano, two tsp.
- Salt to taste
- Olive oil, two tbsp.

Instructions:

1. Take a large bowl and mix all the ingredients together.
2. Now add the olive oil in a baking tray and place the Salmon pieces on it.
3. Bake in a preheated oven at 375 Fahrenheit and roast it.
4. Cut into pieces and serve with grilled vegetables of your choice.
5. You can also serve it along with rice.

11) Slow Roasted Pesto Salmon

Preparation time: 5 minutes

Cooking time: 20 minutes

Serving: 2

Ingredients:

- Basil pesto, four tbsp.
- Salmon fillet, two pounds
- Extra virgin olive oil, one tbsp.

Instructions:

1. Preheat the oven at 375 degrees.
2. Mix all the ingredients together and cover it with an aluminum foil and bake it for 15-20 minutes.
3. Serve it along with roasted vegetables or rice.

12) Baked Halibut

Preparation time: 5 minutes
Cooking time: 20 minutes
Serving: 2
Ingredients:

- Dried oregano, one tsp.
- Halibut fillet, deboned, two pounds
- Extra virgin olive oil, three tbsp.
- Capers, three tbsp.
- Minced garlic, one tbsp.
- White wine, one cup
- Pepper to taste
- Salt to taste

Instructions:

1. Preheat the oven at 375 degrees.
2. Mix all the ingredients together and cover it with an aluminum foil and bake it for 15-20 minutes.
3. Serve it along with roasted vegetables or rice.

13) Fried Cod Fillets

Preparation time: 5 minutes
Cooking time: 20 minutes
Serving: 2
Ingredients:

- Dried oregano, one tsp.
- Cod fillet, deboned, two pounds
- Extra virgin olive oil, three tbsp.
- Capers, three tbsp.
- Minced garlic, one tbsp.
- White wine, one cup
- Pepper to taste
- Salt to taste
- Flour, half cup

Instructions:

1. Marinate the cod fillets by adding all the ingredients together.
2. Now add oil in a deep frying pan and fry the cod fillets by dipping it in flour.
3. Your dish is ready to be served with any dip of your choice.
4. You can also serve it along with rice.

14) Baked Salmon with Fennel and Kalamata Olives

Preparation time: 5 minutes

Cooking time: 20 minutes

Serving: 2

Ingredients:

- Dried oregano, one tsp.
- Salmon fillet, deboned, two pounds
- Extra virgin olive oil, three tbsp.
- Orange juice, three tbsp.
- Minced garlic, one tbsp.
- Fennel bulb, one
- White wine, one cup
- Pepper to taste
- Salt to taste
- Kalamata olives, pitted, half cup
- Bay leaves, two

Instructions:

1. Preheat the oven at 375 degrees.
2. Mix all the ingredients together and cover it with an aluminum foil and bake it for 15-20 minutes.
3. After baking dish, it out and add the olives on top of it.
4. Serve it along with roasted vegetables or rice.

15) Lemon and Parsley Crab Cakes

Preparation time: 15 minutes
Cooking time: 20 minutes
Serving: 2
Ingredients:

- Dijon mustard, half tsp.
- Juice squeezed from half lemon
- Nonstick spray
- Whole wheat bread crumbs, three tbsp.
- Crab meat, 12 oz.
- Parsley, chopped, three tbsp.
- Egg, one
- Cayenne pepper, one tsp.
- Low fat mayonnaise, two tbsp.

Instructions:

1. In a large bowl, add the Dijon mustard, crab meat, cayenne pepper, lemon juice, low fat mayonnaise, parsley, and mix properly.
2. Now make small round shaped balls and dip it in the egg and coat it with bread crumbs.
3. Fry these balls and top with fresh parsley.
4. Your dish is ready to be served.

16) Slow Cooked Turkey Chili

Preparation time: 10 minutes
Cooking time: 8 hours
Serving: 8-10
Ingredients:

- Garlic, minced, half tsp.
- Kidney beans, half cup
- Nonstick spray
- Bell pepper, diced, one
- Turkey meat, two pounds
- Ground cumin, three tbsp.
- Chili powder, three tbsp.
- Dried oregano, one tsp.
- Tomato puree, one cup
- Celery, finely chopped, half cup
- Onions, chopped, half cup
- Water, two cups

Instructions:

1. Add all the ingredients except the turkey in a slow cooker and cook it for 8 hours.
2. Cook the turkey pieces until they turn light brown in color.
3. You can serve it with Greek yoghurt or anything of your choice.
4. Your dish is ready to be served.

17) Slow Cooker Chicken Chili

Preparation time: 10 minutes

Cooking time: 8 hours

Serving: 8-10

Ingredients:

- Garlic, minced, half tsp.
- Kidney beans, half cup
- Nonstick spray
- Bell pepper, diced, one
- Chicken meat, two pounds
- Ground cumin, three tbsp.
- Chili powder, three tbsp.
- Dried oregano, one tsp.
- Tomato puree, one cup
- Celery, finely chopped, half cup
- Onions, chopped, half cup
- Water, two cups

Instructions:

1. Add all the ingredients except the chicken in a slow cooker and cook it for 8 hours.
2. Cook the chicken pieces until they turn light brown in color.
3. You can serve it with Greek yoghurt or anything of your choice.
4. Your dish is ready to be served.

18) Grilled Chicken Wings

Preparation time: 15 minutes
Cooking time: 20 minutes
Serving: 8-10
Ingredients:

- Garlic, minced, half tsp.
- Buffalo wing sauce, one cup
- Extra virgin olive oil, three tbsp.
- Frozen chicken wings, two pounds
- Freshly ground pepper to taste.
- Salt to taste

Instructions:

1. Mix all the ingredients together and cover it for 10 minutes.
2. Now add the olive oil on a grill and place the marinated wings on top.
3. Grill on both sides until crispy and brown in color.
4. Your dish is ready to be served.

The above mentioned lunch recipes are very easy to make and can be followed easily at home.

4.6 Dinner Recipes

This section contains amazing dinner recipes that you can easily follow with the simple instruction in each recipe.

1) Crispy Chicken Tenders

Preparation time: 10 minutes
Cooking time: 20 minutes
Serving: 5-6
Ingredients:

- Garlic, minced, half tsp.
- Dried parsley, one tsp.
- Extra virgin olive oil, three tbsp.
- Frozen chicken tender pieces, two pounds
- Freshly ground pepper to taste.
- Dried dill powder, half tsp.
- Egg, one
- Whole wheat bread crumbs, half cup
- Dried basil, half tsp.
- Dried onion powder, half tsp
- Salt to taste

Instructions:

1. In a large bowl, add the dried dill, dried basil, chicken tenders, dried onion powder, pepper, salt, parsley, and mix properly.
2. Now cover it for 10 minutes.
3. After 10 minutes, dip each tender piece in egg and then the whole wheat bread crumbs.
4. Shallow fry these tender pieces in extra virgin olive oil and top with fresh parsley.
5. Your dish is ready to be served.

2) Chicken Nachos and Sweet Bell Peppers

Preparation time: 10 minutes
Cooking time: 20 minutes
Serving: 5-6
Ingredients:

- Garlic powder, half tsp.
- Tomato, diced, one medium sized
- Extra virgin olive oil, three tbsp.
- Nonstick cooking spray
- Shredded chicken breast, two cups
- Freshly ground pepper to taste.
- Cumin powder, half tsp.
- Shredded cheese, one cup
- Mini bell peppers, one pound
- Paprika, half tsp.
- Onion, minced, half
- Salt to taste
- Black olives, sliced, half cup
- Scallions, for garnishing, chopped
- Jalapeno peppers, few

Instructions:

1. Bake the bell peppers in a preheated oven at 400 Fahrenheit for 10 minutes.
2. In the meanwhile, take a pan and add olive oil, onions, garlic, chicken, tomatoes, cumin powder, paprika, pepper, and salt.
3. Cook it properly.
4. Add the mixture into the mini bell peppers and top it with few olives, cheese, and jalapeno peppers and bake for further ten minutes.
5. Top them with few chopped scallions.
6. Your dish is ready to be served.

3) Creamy Beef Stroganoff and Mushrooms

Preparation time: 10 minutes
Cooking time: 20 minutes
Serving: 2
Ingredients:

- Low fat Greek yoghurt, half cup
- Tomato, diced, one medium sized
- Extra virgin olive oil, three tbsp.
- Nonstick cooking spray
- Beef streaks, extra lean, one pound
- Dried dill, half tsp.
- Water, one cup
- Beef broth, one cup
- Whole wheat flour, two tbsp.
- Dried thyme, half tsp.
- Onion, minced, half
- Salt to taste
- Mushrooms, sliced, half cup
- Worcestershire sauce, one tsp.
- Parsley, half cup, finely chopped

Instructions:

1. Cook the beef streaks in a pan until they turn light brown.
2. Now in another pan, add olive oil, onions and cook for two to three minutes.
3. After a while, add the mushrooms and then add the Worcestershire sauce and cook for a while.
4. Add the water, broth, dried thyme, salt, whole wheat flour, dried dill, tomatoes, and simmer for ten minutes.
5. Now add the yoghurt and keep stirring until dissolved.
6. Add the beef streaks in it and parsley.
7. Your dish is ready to be served.

4) Sloppy Joes

Preparation time: 10 minutes

Cooking time: 20 minutes

Serving: 2

Ingredients:

- Chopped celery, half cup
- Tomato, diced, one medium sized
- Extra virgin olive oil, three tbsp.
- Nonstick cooking spray
- Beef streaks, extra lean, one pound
- Brown sugar, one tbsp.
- Dijon mustard, two tbsp.
- Onion, minced, half
- Salt to taste
- Worcestershire sauce, one tsp.
- Parsley, half cup, finely chopped

Instructions:

1. Cook the beef streaks in a pan until they turn light brown.
2. Now in another pan, add olive oil, onions and cook for two to three minutes.
3. After a while, add the tomatoes and then add the Worcestershire sauce and cook for a while.
4. Add the brown sugar, Dijon mustard, chopped celery, and cook for a few minutes.
5. Add the beef streaks in it and parsley.
6. Your dish is ready to be served.

5) Italian Beef Sandwiches

Preparation time: 10 minutes
Cooking time: 7 hours
Serving: 4
Ingredients:

- Balsamic vinegar, one tbsp.
- Garlic powder, one tsp.
- Onion powder, one tsp.
- Dried oregano, one tsp.
- Beef, extra lean, one pound
- Dried basil, one tsp.
- Onion, chopped, one
- Dried thyme, one tsp.
- Ground pepper, one tsp.
- Salt to taste
- Bread slices, 8-10
- Red bell pepper, sliced, one

Instructions:

1. Add the beef, onion, and bell pepper in a cooker.
2. Add the herbs and spices into the cooker along with water.
3. Cook for 7 hours on slow heat.
4. Slice the beef pieces and place them in the slightly toasted bread.
5. Your dish is ready to be served.

6) Italian Chicken Sandwiches

Preparation time: 10 minutes
Cooking time: 4 hours
Serving: 4
Ingredients:

- Balsamic vinegar, one tbsp.
- Garlic powder, one tsp.
- Onion powder, one tsp.
- Dried oregano, one tsp.
- Chicken breast, extra lean, one pound
- Dried basil, one tsp.
- Onion, chopped, one
- Dried thyme, one tsp.
- Ground pepper, one tsp.
- Salt to taste
- Bread slices, 8-10
- Red bell pepper, sliced, one

Instructions:

1. Add the chicken, onion, and bell pepper in a cooker.
2. Add the herbs and spices into the cooker along with water.
3. Cook for 4 hours on slow heat.
4. Slice the chicken pieces and place them in the slightly toasted bread.
5. You can add any sauce of your choice in it as well.
6. Your dish is ready to be served.

7) Slow Cooker Beef Chili

Preparation time: 10 minutes

Cooking time: 8 hours

Serving: 8-10

Ingredients:

- Garlic, minced, half tsp.
- Kidney beans, half cup
- Nonstick spray
- Bell pepper, diced, one
- Beef meat, two pounds, cut very small
- Ground cumin, three tbsp.
- Chili powder, three tbsp.
- Dried oregano, one tsp.
- Tomato puree, one cup
- Celery, finely chopped, half cup
- Onions, chopped, half cup
- Water, two cups

Instructions:

1. Add all the ingredients except the beef in a slow cooker and cook it for 8 hours.
2. Cook the beef pieces until they turn light brown in color.
3. You can serve it with Greek yoghurt or anything of your choice.
4. Your dish is ready to be served.

8) Baked Beef with Fennel and Asparagus

Preparation time: 5 minutes

Cooking time: 20 minutes

Serving: 2

Ingredients:

- Dried oregano, one tsp.
- Beef, deboned, two pounds
- Extra virgin olive oil, three tbsp.
- Orange juice, three tbsp.
- Minced garlic, one tbsp.
- Fennel bulb, one
- White wine, one cup
- Pepper to taste
- Salt to taste
- Asparagus, half cup
- Bay leaves, two

Instructions:

1. Preheat the oven at 375 degrees.
2. Mix all the ingredients together and cover it with an aluminum foil and bake it for 15-20 minutes.
3. After baking dish it out and add the Roasted asparagus on top of it.
4. Serve it along with roasted vegetables or rice.

9) Broccoli and Cheese Casserole

Preparation time: 10 minutes

Cooking time: 45 minutes

Serving: 6-8

Ingredients:

- Low fat Greek yoghurt, one cup
- Broccoli, partially cooked, two cups, cut into chunks
- Dijon mustard, one tbsp.
- Garlic powder, one tbsp.
- Shredded aged cheddar cheese, one cup
- Shredded mozzarella cheese, half cup

Instructions:

1. Preheat the oven for about 400 Fahrenheit.
2. Mix the yoghurt, garlic powder, Dijon mustard and broccoli together and add it in a baking dish.
3. Top it with cheese and cover it with an aluminum foil. Now, bake it for 35 minutes.
4. Remove the foil and broil it for 10 minutes.
5. Your dish is ready to be served.

10) Fried Chicken Fillets

Preparation time: 5 minutes
Cooking time: 20 minutes
Serving: 2
Ingredients:

- Dried oregano, one tsp.
- Chicken fillet, two pounds
- Extra virgin olive oil, three tbsp.
- Capers, three tbsp.
- Minced garlic, one tbsp.
- White wine, one cup
- Pepper to taste
- Salt to taste
- Flour, half cup

Instructions:

1. Marinate the chicken fillets by adding all the ingredients together.
2. Now add oil in a deep frying pan and fry the cod fillets by dipping it in flour.
3. Your dish is ready to be served with any dip of your choice.
4. You can also serve it along with rice.

11) Lemon and Parsley Chicken Balls

Preparation time: 15 minutes

Cooking time: 20 minutes

Serving: 2

Ingredients:

- Dijon mustard, half tsp.
- Juice squeezed from half lemon
- Nonstick spray
- Whole wheat bread crumbs, three tbsp.
- Chicken meat, 12 oz.
- Parsley, chopped, three tbsp.
- Egg, one
- Cayenne pepper, one tsp.
- Low fat mayonnaise, two tbsp.

Instructions:

1. In a large bowl, add the Dijon mustard, chicken meat, cayenne pepper, lemon juice, low fat mayonnaise, parsley, and mix properly.
2. Now make small round shaped balls and dip it in the egg and coat it with bread crumbs.
3. Fry these balls and top with fresh parsley.
4. Your dish is ready to be served.

12) Chicken Casserole

Preparation time: 10 minutes
Cooking time: 35 minutes
Serving: 6-8
Ingredients:

- Low fat Greek yoghurt, one cup
- Chicken, partially cooked, two cups, cut into chunks
- Dijon mustard, one tbsp.
- Garlic powder, one tbsp.
- Shredded aged cheddar cheese, one cup
- Shredded mozzarella cheese, half cup

Instructions:

1. Preheat the oven for about 400 Fahrenheit.
2. Mix the yoghurt, garlic powder, Dijon mustard, and chicken together and add it in a baking dish.
3. Top it with cheese and cover it with an aluminum foil. Now, bake it for 35 minutes.
4. Remove the foil and broil it for 10 minutes.
5. Your dish is ready to be served.

13) Beef and Bean Casserole

Preparation time: 10 minutes

Cooking time: 35 minutes

Serving: 6-8

Ingredients:

- Low fat Greek yoghurt, one cup
- Beef, partially boiled, two cups, cut into chunks
- Kidney beans, partially boiled, one cup
- Dijon mustard, one tbsp.
- Garlic powder, one tbsp.
- Shredded aged cheddar cheese, one cup
- Shredded mozzarella cheese, half cup

Instructions:

1. Preheat the oven for about 400 Fahrenheit.
2. Mix the yoghurt, garlic powder, kidney beans, Dijon mustard, and boiled beef together and add it in a baking dish.
3. Top it with cheese and cover it with an aluminum foil. Now, bake it for 35 minutes.
4. Remove the foil and broil it for 10 minutes.
5. Your dish is ready to be served.

14) Minced Beef Balls

Preparation time: 15 minutes
Cooking time: 20 minutes
Serving: 2
Ingredients:

- Dijon mustard, half tsp.
- Juice squeezed from half lemon
- Nonstick spray
- Whole wheat bread crumbs, three tbsp.
- Minced beef meat, 12 oz.
- Parsley, chopped, three tbsp.
- Egg, one
- Cayenne pepper, one tsp.
- Low fat mayonnaise, two tbsp.

Instructions:

1. In a large bowl, add the Dijon mustard, minced beef, cayenne pepper, lemon juice, low fat mayonnaise, parsley, and mix properly.
2. Now make small round shaped balls and dip it in the egg and coat it with bread crumbs.
3. Fry these balls and top with fresh parsley.
4. Your dish is ready to be served.

15) Baked Chicken with Mix Vegetables

Preparation time: 5 minutes
Cooking time: 20 minutes
Serving: 2
Ingredients:

- Dried oregano, one tsp.
- Chicken breast, two pounds
- Extra virgin olive oil, three tbsp.
- Orange juice, three tbsp.
- Minced garlic, one tbsp.
- Fennel bulb, one
- White wine, one cup
- Pepper to taste
- Salt to taste
- Asparagus, half cup
- Carrots, half cup
- Potatoes, half cup
- Bay leaves, two

Instructions:

1. Preheat the oven at 375 degrees.
2. Mix all the ingredients together and cover it with an aluminum foil and bake it for 15-20 minutes.
3. After baking dish, it out and add the roasted carrots, potatoes and asparagus on top of it.
4. Serve it along with roasted vegetables or rice.

16) Chicken and Mushroom Risotto

Preparation time: 5 minutes

Cooking time: 55 minutes

Serving: 6

Ingredients:

- Garlic, minced, one tsp.
- Leaks, diced, two
- Extra virgin olive oil, one tbsp.
- Sliced mushrooms, four cups
- Fresh spinach leaves, three cups
- White wine, half cup
- Chicken broth, one cup
- Chicken pieces, small, one cup
- Thyme, two tsp.

Instructions:

1. In a large deep pan, add the olive oil and garlic. Cook it for a few seconds and add the leeks and mushrooms.
2. Add the barley and thyme and cook for a few minutes.
3. Add the wine and mix it properly.
4. Add the broth and let it simmer for 30 minutes on low heat.
5. Now add the spinach and mix till they are wilted.
6. Your dish is ready to be served.

17) Minced Beef and Spaghetti Squash Casserole

Preparation time: 10 minutes
Cooking time: 35 minutes
Serving: 6-8
Ingredients:

- Low fat Greek yoghurt, one cup
- Minced beef, partially cooked, two cups, cut into chunks
- Dijon mustard, one tbsp.
- Garlic powder, one tbsp.
- Spaghetti squash, 3 pounds
- Shredded aged cheddar cheese, one cup
- Shredded mozzarella cheese, half cup

Instructions:

1. Preheat the oven for about 400 Fahrenheit.
2. Bake the Spaghetti squash for 10 minutes and then use a fork to make the spaghetti structure from the inner material and throw out the skin
3. Mix the yoghurt, garlic powder, Dijon mustard, spaghetti squash, minced beef together, and add it in a baking dish.
4. Top it with cheese and cover it with an aluminum foil. Now, bake it for 25 minutes.
5. Remove the foil and broil it for 10 minutes.
6. Your dish is ready to be served.

18) Coconut and Chicken Curry

Preparation time: 15 minutes

Cooking time: 30 minutes

Serving: 6

Ingredients:

- Grated ginger, one tbsp.
- Minced garlic, one tbsp.
- Cinnamon, quarter tsp.
- Turmeric, half tsp.
- Curry powder, two tsp.
- Ground cumin, half tsp.
- Coconut oil, three tbsp.
- Chicken pieces, 14 oz.
- Unsweetened coconut milk, two cups
- Tomato puree, one cup
- Carrots, diced, two
- Bok Choi, two stems
- Chicken broth, two cups
- Fresh cilantro, half cup

Instructions:

1. Cook the chicken cubes in the coconut oil for 3-4 minutes till a firm layer forms on the chicken cubes
2. Add the rest of the ingredients by first removing the tofu from the pan.
3. Mix the coconut milk into it. Now add the tofu and bok choi into the mixture and cook it for few minutes.
4. Serve it with rice and garnish it with fresh cilantro.

19) Garlic and Herb Grilled Beef

Preparation time: 10 minutes
Cooking time: 25 minutes
Serving: 2
Ingredients:
- Low fat Greek yoghurt, one cup
- Beef Steak, two pounds
- Dijon mustard, one tbsp.
- Garlic powder, one tbsp.
- Dried basil, one tsp.
- Dried thyme, one tsp.
- Dried dill, one tsp.
- Dried oregano, one tsp.
- Salt to taste
- Olive oil, two tbsp.

Instructions:
1. Take a large bowl and mix all the ingredients together.
2. Now add the olive oil on a grill and place the beef steaks on it.
3. Cook on each side.
4. Cut into pieces and serve with grilled vegetables of your choice.
5. You can also serve it along with rice.

The above mentioned 100 different recipes of smoothies, salads, broths and soups, and various recipes for breakfast, lunch, and dinners can be followed easily at home.

Chapter 5: Keeping Yourself Healthy and Motivated

Undergoing a surgery and following a diet plan is not enough for reducing weight and keeping yourself healthy. All the hard work can go in vain if you are not motivated towards your goal. You can easily lose your tract of being conscious and passionate about your health so, it is very important to keep yourself motivated. In this chapter, you will get the different tips of keeping yourself motivated and focused as well as the different techniques to lead a sound and healthy life.

5.1 Tips on Keeping Yourself Motivated

Keeping yourself motivated after a gastric sleeve surgery to reduce further weight and perform exercise can be very tricky and difficult. You can use the following tips to keep your motivation intact:

- Numerous individuals get fit stall out with regards to where they need to be and when they should stop after gastric sleeve medical procedure. The risk that one can put themselves at with this is of getting underweight or anorexic. It can become like a race to get down to objective weight, yet then they do not have a clue how to quit losing and stick inside range. Some basic advances that you can do to guarantee you do not put yourself in danger of being underweight are to ascertain your optimal weight territory. Stick with around a 10-pound range that you permit yourself to remain between, for example, 150 to 160 pounds. At the point when you permit yourself a range, you remove a ton of the pressure of hitting a precise number, and you know not to drop down underneath that run as it is beneficial to stay within it.

- At the point when you begin to slip on what are solid propensities, try giving motivational speeches yourself to refocus. You cannot generally have someone there to take you to the rec center, cook your nourishments for you, or remind you to take your nutrients. In the event that you begin tumbling off course, do not excuse it and let yourself think it is alright, or you will slip into a perilous pattern of defending helpless practices. Similarly, if you at that point where you go on vacation for a couple of days, which turns into a couple of more weeks, a month, past a month. You are going to go again; however, then perhaps some family gives come up, your back damages, or you have a migraine. These things keep coming up, and you let them prevent you from getting out and being dynamic. It is significant that you build up a sound mental demeanor and accomplish something by bouncing up, grin into the mirror, and stately "I am going to go for a run." You will be amazed at how great you will feel after that and how you will shockingly have the vitality you had previously figured you did not have. This equivalent attitude becomes possibly the most important factor with diet and different everyday issues too. Always keep in mind that gastric sleeve medical procedure is more a device than a total weight reduction arrangement.

- Some get all energized from the outset and need to get in shape as fast as could be expected under the circumstances. Thus they drop a few pounds until they arrive at their objective just to find that they do not have the foggiest idea what to do from that point. This occasionally prompts getting into negative behavior patterns and falling right back to where they were before they experienced gastric sleeve medical procedure in any case. The way to taking care of this issue is to understand that being solid is a basic framework, not a race to be won.

- After experiencing gastric sleeve medical procedure, numerous patients find that it gets exhausting to eat similar stuff, drink similar protein drinks, and go on the same walk or do a similar exercise schedule. However, it does not mean you have to eat similar nourishments or do similar activities constantly. Switch things up by concocting new plans to attempt through some accommodating sites. The equivalent goes for practices you do to keep yourself dynamic every day. You do not need to lift loads or run to be dynamic as those are only some famously advertised strategies for keeping genuinely dynamic. You can do yoga, pilates, tennis, ball, swimming, full-body cardio, and significantly more. However, if you cannot escape the house to go for a work out session, you can even go to YouTube and type in-home full-body cardio, gastric sleeve works out, etc.

- One terrible propensity that should be halted for some individuals is keeping some snacks and fat dense foods away from visual perception and simple reach in the kitchen. You return home in the wake of a tough day at work and advantageously have a pack of chips, jellies, perhaps some treats in that spot for you to get off the counter and enjoy. So what would you be able to do to cure this issue? The appropriate response is just to throw away or lose the shoddy nourishment with the goal that you do not have the enticement gazing you in the face. If you cannot get the nourishments out of your home because of relatives or the craving to sometimes treat yourself, that is completely fine. Simply conceal the food where you will not see it often, for example, over your refrigerator or at the head of your wash room above eye level. At that point, place sound nourishments out where you see them promptly and at eye level in the wash room. So as opposed to snatching those chips or that sweet treat, you can get some blended nuts, baby carrots, possibly some apple cuts. This will assist you in keeping your body better sustained since these

130

nourishments contain nutrients, fiber, and minerals that your body needs.

- Ensure that you discover somebody who will get down on you about your helpless decisions or terrible practices. That individual will assist you with remaining on target and assist you with pushing ahead with your weight reduction and weight upkeep plan. In the event that you get an empowering influence as a responsibility accomplice, you may not end up stuck at a weight recapture. This is an opportunity to be straightforward with yourself and to be overly legitimate about your examples of conduct considering your wellbeing.

- Compose the solid feast plan, get the nutritious food, go for an exercise, and continue doing it again and again. The demonstration of rehearsing an action, again and again, makes it easy after some time since you become accustomed to doing it. On the first occasion, when you do anything, it is supposed to be troublesome. The more you make a move, the simpler it will get. Likewise, as the weight falls off, you will feel better moving in your body on the grounds that there will be less to carry around.

- You can be the cause of all your own problems when glancing in the mirror. Quiet your inward pundit and have a go at rehashing positive certifications to yourself consistently. Additionally, abstain from contrasting yourself with others. Keep in mind that each weight reduction venture is unique.

- There is a particular outcome that individuals need from making a move. This is likewise why inspiration is connected with defining and accomplishing objectives. If by chance somebody accepts that it will take a ton of hard, predictable work to get to a particular outcome, they will probably

131

maintain a strategic distance from the assignment and have low inspiration as a result of the envisioned or saw torment included (enthusiastic, physical, mental, and so on.) in getting to their ideal outcome or objective. So, as expected, they dawdle, and later, the errand feels greater, and thus, they accept they have low or no inspiration. So, in short, always consider your tasks easy to be achieved so you can get to your goal quickly.

- Your weight reduction medical procedure is a viable method to lose abundance weight; however, it is anything but a marvel fix. You may hit a weight reduction level or recapture a little weight, yet do not let this perplex you. Be prepared for potential difficulties, and keep looking forward.

- Figure out how to give yourself a somewhat congratulatory gesture. Prize yourself with something pleasant like a back rub or a long shower. Make a point to maintain a strategic distance from any food-related prizes since that could prompt undesirable propensities.

- Try not to race into a high power exercise and anticipate quick outcomes, as that may prompt disappointment. After your medical procedure, you will have to take things moderate with regard to your eating routine and physical movement levels. Simplicity into an agreeable schedule that fits with your way of life.

- Ensure that your home and your environmental factors are helpful for your new way of life. Dispose of any enticing nourishments, and fill the wash room with more beneficial alternatives. Additionally, have a go at keeping your tennis shoes by the entryway to remind you to work out.

- By straightforwardly following your medical procedure, you will get in shape quickly; however, in the long run, this will back off. Show restraint toward yourself, set aside some effort to understand that your weight reduction medical procedure and way of life changes for wellbeing are a long lasting responsibility to a superior and more advantageous you.

After weight reduction medical procedure, there will be days while staying cheery and spurred will be hard. Your weight reduction medical procedure is the start of your excursion to a more beneficial life, so continue pushing ahead by making plans to discover things that make you cheerful and inspire you to be effective.

5.2 Leading a Sound and Healthy Life after the Surgery

The vast majority accept that the activity just powers individuals to eat less by making their stomachs very small. Yet, researchers have found that it really causes significant changes in a patient's physiology, modifying the movement of thousands of qualities in the human body just as the complex hormonal motioning from the gut to the brain. It regularly prompts bewildering changes in the manner things taste; making desires for a rich cut of chocolate cake or a sack of burgers essentially disappear. The individuals who have the medical procedure normally settle at a lower weight.

Bariatric medical procedure, strategies to instigate weight reduction, which makes a little stomach pocket; sleeve gastrectomy, which diminishes the stomach to 25 percent of its size; lap band medical procedure, in which a gadget is set around the stomach to hinder eating; and duodenal switch medical procedure, in which 70 percent of the stomach is evacuated and a huge segment of the small digestive system is rerouted. All of these medical procedures have a similar objective: to enable seriously hefty patients to get thinner

133

rapidly and adequately by confining the amount they can eat just as what number of calories they assimilate. Bariatric medical procedure likewise enables fat patients to control their related conditions, for example, diabetes, hypertension, and rest apnea.

Tumors are connected to corpulence—particularly colon, bosom, and endometrial malignant growths. We do not have long haul studies to show that individuals who have been large for a long time, and afterward have weight reduction medical procedure, will have a lower chance. In any case, we accept that working prior (and keep individuals less fatty for a long time) will lessen these malignant growth dangers.

Bariatric medical procedure patients likewise have fewer hospitalizations, shorter emergency clinic stays, and are less inclined to be admitted to the emergency unit. That is contrasted with hefty patients who do not have a bariatric medical procedure. Studies show that higher levels of bariatric patients are alive, contrasted with the individuals who did not have a medical procedure. We have additionally observed enhancements in ladies with polycystic ovary maladies, barrenness, ulcers, leg growth. Each time we pivot, we discover wellbeing upgrades. For some patients, it's a hazard they are willing to take. Here and there, the more wiped out you are as a result of your weight, the greater the advantage of having the medical procedure. A Bariatric medical procedure will get you closer to your life objectives.

Conclusion

Weight reduction procedures have been in fashion since the past decade, and everyone seems to be adopting them. Gastric bariatric sleeve surgery has been known as an operating treatment to cut off weight from your body by removing 75% of your stomach. In this way you feel less hungry and achieve satiety quite easily. Sleeve surgery can be a success and an achievement for those patients with a BMI higher than 30.

In this book, you were given an overview of everything related to gastric bariatric sleeve surgery, starting up with what actually is this surgery and how does it work. Surgeries can be really frightening for some individuals, so keeping them confident can be quite a hectic task. There are various advantages and benefits of gastric sleeve surgery that are discussed in the first chapter. You can prepare for your surgery in advance with the amazing tips that are mentioned in the chapter.

There are several factors that need consideration before undergoing a procedure, many people may experience this procedure without the consultation of their health specialist and may regret later on. The process of recovering from a surgery involves many things, so in the second chapter, you are given many wonderful tips and techniques to recover quickly from the surgery without any hindrance.

This book covered 100 different recipes that include smoothies, broths, and salads. Recipes for breakfast, lunch, and dinners are also mentioned with easy to follow instructions so you can formulate them on your own. You can follow these amazing recipes and continue to lose more weight after the surgery. You can create your own diet plan by focusing on the salient points mentioned in the book; following these guidelines is a must after the surgery for quick recovery and effective weight loss. A therapeutic diet for 30 days is also mentioned in the book, which you can easily follow by keeping the calorie count intact. Likewise, you can even make the diet plan yourself by adding any recipe from the ones added in the book.

In the end, having a surgery or following a specific diet plan is never enough if you are not focused or motivated towards your goal. It is very important to keep yourself motivated at all times, follow the easy tips mentioned in the last chapter. Leading a healthy and sound life is not at all difficult once you start shedding the extra weight your body is carrying.

Part 2

Introduction

Thank you for doing so.

The following chapters will discuss many recipes that can change the way you prepare your meals. You will want to maintain a good weight loss program. Each one of these meals has all the essential information to incorporate them into your new way of life.

There are plenty of books on this subject on the market, thanks again for choosing this one! Every effort was made to ensure it is full of as much useful information as possible. Please enjoy!

Chapter 1: Breakfast Goodies

Crustless Quiche

Servings: 6
Calories: 106.8
Prep and Cooking Time: 00:50:00

Ingredients
2 c egg beaters/egg whites
1 c cottage cheese (non-fat)
½ c each:
Chopped – cooked broccoli
Diced lean ham
Colby or cheddar shredded cheese
Cooking spray
Pepper and salt to taste

Instructions
1. Set the oven temperature to 375ºF. Spray a casserole dish with the cooking spray and add all of the ingredients.
2. Bake until the center is set (45 minutes).

Sausage and Mushroom Gravy

Servings: 4
Calories: 115.4
Prep and Cooking Time: 00:17

Ingredients
8 ounces/2 c chopped mushrooms**
¼ large chopped onions
2 tbsp each:
Olive oil
Whole wheat flour
¼ tsp each:
Black pepper
Red pepper flakes
Dried sage
½ tsp dried thyme
1 ½ c skim milk
**For best results use the white button or baby bella mushrooms.

Instructions
1. Place the oil and onions in a sauté pan. After two minutes, toss in the mushrooms and continue cooking another three to four minutes.
2. Fold in the flour, mixing for one minute, and combine with the spices.
3. Gently, empty in the milk, stirring until the sauce is creamy. Simmer about five more minutes

Eggs

Baked Egg Cups

Servings: 6
Calories: 125.6
Prep and Cooking Time: 00:30:00

Ingredients
6 eggs
6 slices deli ham – lean
½ c 2% cheddar cheese – shredded
1 tbsp chopped chives
Pepper
Non-stick cooking spray

Instructions
1. Set the oven temperature at 350ºF.
2. Lightly spray six muffin tins and arrange the ham slices to line the cup. Bake ten minutes.
3. Take the tins out of the oven and add an egg to each cup.
4. Break the yolk and add a sprinkle of pepper.
5. Bake another ten minutes if they are done to your preference. Garnish with cheese and chives.

Egg in a Basket

Servings: 1
Calories: 246.2
Prep and Cooking Time: 00:15

Ingredients
1 large egg
1 slice of bread
Butter flavored cooking spray

Instructions
1. Remove the middle out of the slice of bread using a glass.
2. Use some cooking spray on a griddle with the medium heat setting.
3. Arrange the bread on the skillet/griddle and add the broken egg.
4. Cook until done.

Eggs and Oats

Servings: 1
Calories: 272.6
Prep and Cooking Time: 00:10:00

Ingredients

2 egg whites
1 whole egg
2 ounces skim milk
½ c rolled oats (Quaker)
Optional Garnishes:
Hot sauce
Cayenne

Honey cinnamon berries

Instructions

1. Use some non-stick cooking spray to lightly grease a skillet. Add all of the ingredients.
2. Cook as with any scrambled egg.

Sausage and Egg Casserole

Servings: 12
Calories: 200.5
Prep and Cooking Time: 00:40

Ingredients
12 large eggs
¼ c skim milk
12 ounces breakfast sausage – browned
¼ tsp pepper
2 c low-fat cheddar shredded cheese

Instructions
1. Program the oven temperature to 375ºF.
2. Mix all of the components and empty the mixture into a lightly greased 12-c muffin pan.
3. Bake 30 minutes, cool for five, and serve.

Note: This can also be baked in a casserole dish.

Spinach and Feta Egg Whites

Servings: 1
Calories: 200.3
Prep and Cooking Time: 00:15:00

Ingredients
2 c baby spinach
3 egg whites
1 chopped tomato
¼ c each:
Chopped onion
Crumbled feta cheese

Instructions
1. Chop the veggies and add them in a pan to cook using medium heat, cooking the onions until they are translucent.
2. Add the spinach, tomato, and egg whites. Blend in the ½ of the cheese.
3. Garnish the top with the remainder of cheese, pepper, and salt.

Muffins and Breakfast Cookies

Blueberry Muffin

Servings: 12
Calories: 102.8
Prep and Cooking Time: 00:35

Ingredients
½ tsp. salt
1 c of each:
Flour

Old-fashioned oats
1 tsp. each:
Baking soda
Cinnamon

½ c each:
Unsweetened applesauce
Water

Sugar

2 egg whites
1 c frozen blueberries

Instructions
1. Prepare 12 muffin tins and program the oven to 350ºF.
2. Combine the salt, soda, cinnamon, oats, and flour.
3. Add the egg whites, sugar, water, and applesauce.
4. Blend in the blueberries.
5. Bake until lightly browned or about 20-25 minutes

Bran, Flaxseed, and Wheat Muffins

Servings: 24
Calories: 115.7
Prep and Cooking Time: 00:45:00

Ingredients
1 c of each:
Ground flaxseed
Brown sugar
Oat bran
Whole wheat flour
2 tsp. baking soda
2 tbsp cinnamon
1 tsp. baking powder
½ tsp. salt
1 ½ - c shredded carrots
2-3 apples
½ tsp. salt
¾ c 2% milk
2 beaten eggs
1 tsp. vanilla
½ c each (**Optional**):
Raisins

Chopped nuts

Instructions
1. Prepare 24 paper liners/oil lined muffin tin. Set the oven to 350ºF.
2. Core and chop the apples.
3. Blend the sugar, bran, flaxseed, flour, and other dry ingredients.
4. Shred the apples and carrots and toss with the nuts and raisins and all dry ingredients.

5. Whip the eggs, milk, and vanilla. Blend into the dry mixture.
6. Fill each cup ¾ full. Bake for 20 to 25 minutes.

Healthy Breakfast Cookie

Servings: 30
Calories: 111.1
Prep and Cooking Time: 00:30

Ingredients
2 large eggs
¼ c butter
½ c each:
Honey

Chopped - dried apricots
Raisins

1 c of each:
Grated carrots
Chopped walnuts
Rolled oats
All-purpose flour
1 ½ c Cheerios
1 tsp. each:
Nutmeg
Cinnamon

Instructions
1. Combine the egg, butter, and honey in a mixing dish. Blend in the apricots, walnuts, and raisins.
2. In a separate container, mix the cinnamon, nutmeg, flour, and oats.
3. Combine all components and add the Cheerios.
4. Drop the mixture/dough onto a baking sheet about one inch apart.
5. Bake 15 minutes or until the cookie is firm.

Pumpkin Muffins

Servings: 18
Calories: 340
Prep and Cooking Time: 00:35:00

Ingredients
1 can (1 pound) pumpkin
1 box spice cake mix
½ c flaxseed meal

Instructions
1. Program the temperature in the oven to 350ºF.
2. Prepare a muffin tin with paper liners or cooking spray.
3. Combine all of the ingredients and bake 25 minutes.

Zucchini Bread Muffins

Servings: 24
Calories: 139.6
Prep and Cooking Time: 00:50

Ingredients
3 large egg whites
2 c of each:
Sugar

Grated zucchini
1 c applesauce
1 tbsp vanilla
½ tsp salt
2 tsp baking powder
3 c whole wheat flour
1 tsp baking soda
3 tsp brown sugar
2 tsp cinnamon

Instructions
1. Set the oven temperature to 350ºF.
2. Grease 24 muffin tins with some non-stick cooking spray.
3. Combine the sugar and eggs along with the applesauce, vanilla, and zucchini.
4. Slowly, add the dry components. Mix well.
5. Empty the batter and sprinkle each one with a pinch of brown sugar.
6. Bake 20-30 minutes.

Oatmeal Dishes

Banana – Peanut Butter Oatmeal

Servings: 1
Calories: 203.5
Prep and Cooking Time: 00:05:00

Ingredients
½ tbsp creamy peanut butter
¼ c each:
Quick-cooking oats
Skim milk
½ of a large banana

Instructions
1. Peel and slice the banana; puree.
2. Pour the oatmeal and banana into a dish. Stir and cook for 30 seconds on high, uncovered in the microwave.
3. Stir the mixture again, and cook another 30 seconds.
4. Blend in the peanut butter.

Blue Oatmeal

Servings: 2
Calories: 214.2
Prep and Cooking Time: 00:10

Ingredients
2 tbsp flaxseed (ground flax)
1 c 100% natural whole grain oatmeal
2 tsp brown sugar
1 ½ - c water
½ tbsp unsweetened dry cocoa powder
½ c frozen - unsweetened blueberries

Instructions
1. Bring the water to boiling and dump the dry fixings into a saucepan.
2. Lower the heat and cook two to three minutes on low heat.
3. Stir in the frozen berries and enjoy.

Pumpkin Pie Oatmeal

Servings: 2
Calories: 164.2
Prep and Cooking Time: 00:25:00

Ingredients
1 c non-fat milk
½ c each:
Canned pumpkin
Uncooked old-fashioned oatmeal
¼ tsp pumpkin pie spice
Pinch of ground cardamom
1 tbsp sugar

Instructions
1. Mix all of the ingredients listed and cook until thick; usually about 20 minutes.

Slow Cooker 6 – Grain Breakfast

Servings: 4
Calories: 134.5
Prep and Cooking Time: 8:05

Ingredients
¼ c rolled oats
2 ½ tbsp each:
Brown rice
Bulgur wheat
Quinoa

Barley

1 c diced apples
3 c water
1 ½ tsp ground cinnamon
1 tbsp vanilla extract

Instructions
1. Mix all of the fixings in the slow cooker.
2. Set the cooker on the low setting for six to eight hours.
3. Stir and add small amounts of water if desired.

Summertime Uncooked Oatmeal

Servings: 1
Calories: 391.3
Prep and Cooking Time: 00:05:00

Ingredients
About 25 raisins
½ c each:
Milk

Oats

1 tsp cinnamon

Instructions
1. Thoroughly blend each the ingredients in a covered dish and place them in the refrigerator overnight.
2. Enjoy the next morning without any cooking.

Pancakes and Waffles

Banana Bread Pancakes

Servings: 8
Calories: 126.2
Prep and Cooking Time: 00:30

Ingredients
2 pouches Quaker Instant Oatmeal – Banana Bread – weight control
2/3 c cottage cheese
2 eggs or ½ c egg beaters
Garnish: Cinnamon and vanilla extract

Instructions
1. Combine all of the components for the pancakes into a blender.
2. Cook over med-high setting on the stovetop.
3. Make 8 (6 inch) pancakes and enjoy.

Cheesecake Pancakes

Servings: 2
Calories: 293.5
Prep and Cooking Time: 00:20:00

Ingredients

4 ounces cream cheese
2 large eggs
Splenda to taste
1 tbsp flaxseed
½ tsp ground cinnamon

Instructions

1. Whisk the egg whites into stiff peaks.
2. Drop the cream cheese into a bowl and blend with the mixer until smooth. Combine this with the yolks and sweetener, flaxseed meal, salt, and cinnamon. Fold in the whipped eggs.
3. Using med-low heat, lightly grease a frying pan.
4. Use ¼ c per pancake and cook for two to three minutes per side.

Cinnamon Pancakes

Servings: 8
Calories: 92.6
Prep and Cooking Time: 00:50-01:00

Ingredients
1 ¼ - c whole wheat flour
1 tsp. baking soda
2 tbsp each:
Splenda

Cinnamon

1 tbsp vanilla extract
½ c egg beaters
1 c skim milk

Instructions
1. Combine the baking soda, flour, and Splenda in a mixing dish.
2. In another dish, blend the vanilla, milk, and eggs. Blend it into the dry ingredients (step 1). Add the cinnamon last.
3. Pour the batter into the pan 1/3 c for each pancake.

Cottage Cheese and Oatmeal Pancakes

Servings: 6
Calories: 47.5
Prep and Cooking Time: 00:40:00 to 00:45:00

Ingredients
4 egg whites
1-2 packets Stevia
½ c each:
Dry oatmeal
Fat-free cottage cheese
½ tsp each:
Vanilla
Baking powder

Instructions
1. Add all of the ingredients into a blender except for the oats. When the mixture is smooth, slowly pour in the oats.
2. Add berries if you like, but add them after the mixture is blended.
3. Cook the pancakes until done and top with your favorite sugar-free syrup.

Oatmeal Pancakes

Servings: 4
Calories: 271.3
Prep and Cooking Time:00:35

Ingredients
1 ¼ c each:
Old Fashioned Quaker Oats
Skim milk
1 large egg
1 tbsp light olive oil
1 tsp baking powder
1 c whole wheat flour

Instructions
1. Mix the milk and oats in a medium dish and let them set for five minutes.
2. Add the oil and egg. Mix and add the dry ingredients.
3. Add the batter (¼ c portions) onto a lightly greased skillet. Cook until browned. Flip over and cook until done.
4. Top it off with some yogurt, maple syrup, preserves or others (not counted in nutritional counts).

Whole Wheat Applesauce Pancakes

Servings: 4
Calories: 188.3
Prep and Cooking Time: 00:35:00

Ingredients
1 ¼ - c. whole wheat flour
2 tsp. baking powder
9 tsp. artificial sweetener/2 tbsp sugar
½ tsp. salt
2 tbsp applesauce
1 c. skim milk
1 beaten egg

Instructions
1. Whisk all of the fixings together and cook on a hot skillet.
2. Serve and enjoy!

Sweets for Breakfast

Flax and Fruit Smoothie

Servings: 1
Calories: 428.9
Prep Time: 00:10

Ingredients
½ - 1 c water
1 scoop low-carb protein powder plain/vanilla
½ c coconut milk
1/3 c frozen strawberries/favorite
2 tbsp flaxseed meal
Splenda/stevia – no carbs

Instructions
1. Combine all of the ingredients in your blender.
2. Serve right away and enjoy

Mixed Berry Smoothie

Servings: 2
Calories: 257.8
Prep Time: 00:10

Ingredients
1 c of each:
Skim milk
Fat-free yogurt
¾ c frozen assorted berries/your choice
Optional: ¼ c sugar

Instructions
1. Empty the yogurt and milk into a blender along with the berries.
2. Add some protein powder if you choose and enjoy.

Servings: 2

Calories: 257.8| Protein: 11.1 g | Fat: 2.8 g | Carbohydrates: 47.4 g

Mocha Banana Smoothie

Servings: 2
Calories: 170.5
Prep Time: 1:10

Ingredients
1 medium banana
1 c fat-free milk
1-2 tbsp honey/sugar
2 tbsp - instant - coffee crystals
1 tbsp unsweetened cocoa powder
½ tsp vanilla
1 c crushed ice/small cubes

Instructions
1. Freeze the banana for one hour and slice into ½ inch slices.
2. Combine all of the goodies in a blender, adding the ice last.
3. Enjoy when smooth.

Strawberry Smoothie

Servings: 2
Calories: 50
Prep Time: 00:10

-

Ingredients

8 ounces low-fat strawberry yogurt
2 c frozen strawberries
¾ c milk

Instructions

1. Blend all of the nutritious components and enjoy.

Yogurt Breakfast Popsicles

Servings: 6
Calories: 75
Prep Time: 04:10

Ingredients
½ c each:
Instant/regular oats
Skim/1% milk
1 c of each:
Greek yogurt - non-fat plain
Chopped fruits/mixed berries
Also Needed: Popsicle molds

Instructions
1. Combine the yogurt and milk and pour into two molds.
2. Add a few berries to each one along with half of the oatmeal.
3. Add an ice cream stick to each mold and freeze for a minimum of four hours.

Chapter 2: Salads and Sandwiches

Caprese Salad

Servings: **2**
Calories: 375
Prep Time: 00:10

Ingredients
6 ounces strawberries
1 ripe avocado
1 (7 ounces) sliced mozzarella ball
Small handful salad leaves
2-3 tbsp balsamic dressing – your choice
Pepper and salt

Instructions
1. Toss in the salad leaves, avocado, strawberries, and cheese into a serving dish.
2. Garnish with the dressing and sprinkle with the pepper and salt. Gently toss.

California Roll in a Bowl

Servings: 4
Calories: 199.1
Prep Time: 00:15

Ingredients
1 head chopped lettuce
1 c cooked brown rice
1 English cucumber – seedless – thinly sliced
1 (8 ounces) package cooked shrimp/crabmeat – chopped
1 grated carrot
1 ripe diced avocado
3 tbsp pickled ginger

For the Dressing
1 tbsp light soy sauce
½ tsp wasabi powder – to taste
3 tbsp rice wine vinegar
Garnishes:
1 large sheet seaweed/nori (toasted and in small bits)
1 tbsp sesame seeds

Instructions
1. Combine all of the fixings for the dressing in a bowl and whisk well.
2. Divide it into four sections and enjoy.

Note: You can locate the ginger in the Asian section of the supermarket.

Caramel Apple Salad

Servings: 16
Calories: 90.7
Prep Time: 00:10

Ingredients

1 box butterscotch pudding mix (sugar-free instant)
1 tub (8 ounces) Cool Whip Free
1 can (14 ounces) pineapple tidbits with the juice
4 large each:
Fuji apples/Red Delicious
Granny Smith apples

Instructions

1. Mix the pineapple with its juice and the pudding mix in a large mixing container.
2. Dice the apples into small bits and combine with the mixture.
3. Fold in the Cool Whip, mix well, and chill.

Chickpea and Feta Salad

Servings: 1
Calories: 285.2
Prep Time: 00:15

Ingredients

¾ c chopped raw vegetables
¼ c each:
Can/fresh chickpeas
Crumbled feta cheese
1 tsp dried oregano
2 tbsp olive oil
1 tbsp lemon juice
Dash each of:
Salt
Pepper

Instructions

1. Use your imagination for the chopped veggies. Include peppers, avocado, tomatoes, onions, and celery or your favorites.
2. Rinse and drain the chickpeas.
3. Combine all of the ingredients and keep it chilled in the fridge until ready to serve.

Coleslaw

Servings: 6
Calories: 71.7
Prep Time: 00:15

Ingredients
1 small shredded carrot
3 c green cabbage – shredded
¼ c minced onion
1 tbsp vinegar
1/3 c mayonnaise
2 tsp sugar
½ tsp each:
Celery seed
Salt

Instructions
1. Prepare the onion, carrots, and cabbage into a bowl.
2. Mix the dressing and pour over the slaw.

Cucumber and Onion Salad with Vinegar

Servings: 6
Calories: 67.5
Prep Time:00:10

Ingredients
Pinch of salt and pepper
1 red onion
3-5 cucumbers (peeled)
½ c each:
White vinegar
Water

1/3 c sugar

Instructions
1. Slice the cucumbers and onions very thin and add to a salad dish.
2. Combine the water, vinegar, salt, pepper, and sugar and pour over the veggies.
3. Add a cover and marinate for a minimum of one hour.

Egg Salad

Servings: **6**
Calories: 115.7
Prep Time: 00:20

Ingredients
3 celery stalks
6 large hard-boiled eggs
2 tbsp pickle relish
¼ c of each:
Diced onions
Reduced fat mayonnaise

Optional:
Pepper

1 tsp mustard
Dash of each:
Celery seed
Paprika

Instructions
1. Peel and chop the eggs, celery, and onions.
2. Combine all of the fixings and chill in the refrigerator until ready for your meal.

Grape Salad

Servings: 16
Calories: 133.7
Prep Time: 01:30

Ingredients

2-4 pounds of grapes (green, red, or both)
1 package of fat-free– 8 ounces each:
Sour cream
Softened cream cheese
½ c each:
Splenda/your choice
Walnuts/pecans

¼ c brown sugar
4 tbsp vanilla extract

Instructions

1. Wash and drain the grapes.
2. Combine the sour cream, cream cheese, vanilla, and sugar—blending well for about three to four minutes on high with a mixer.
3. Toss in the grapes and toss until covered.
4. Bake in a 9x13 cake pan. Sprinkle lightly with the brown sugar. Add the nuts.
5. Chill about one hour before serving.

Israeli Salad

Servings: 8
Calories: 65.2
Prep Time: 00:10

Ingredients
1 medium peeled cucumber
3 medium tomatoes
1 yellow/green bell pepper
3 tbsp. extra-virgin olive oil
2 tbsp. lemon juice
1 tsp. of each: Salt and pepper

Instructions
1. Dice all of the veggies and combine the rest of the ingredients.

Sunshine Fruit Salad

Servings: 10
Calories: 135.2
Prep Time: 01:10

Ingredients

2 cans (15 ounces each) mandarin oranges in light syrup
3 cans (20 ounces each) pineapple chunks in 100% juice
2 large bananas
3 medium kiwi fruits – bite-sized

Instructions

1. Drain the oranges and pineapple. Reserve the pineapple juice.
2. Combine all of the fruit (omit the bananas).
3. Submerge the fruit with the juice and chill for a minimum of one hour.
4. Slice and stir in the bananas before serving.

Sandwiches

Apple and Tuna Sandwich

Servings: 3
Calories: 250
Prep Time: 00:15

Ingredients
1 diced apple
1 can (6.5ounces) packed in water – drained
½ tsp honey
1 tsp mustard
¼ c low-fat vanilla yogurt
3 lettuce leaves
6 slices whole wheat bread

Instructions
1. Wash, peel, and chop the apple.
2. Remove the water from the tuna and combine with the apple, honey, mustard, and yogurt in a mixing dish. Blend well.
3. Add the mixture to three slices of bread. Add the lettuce and the other slice of bread.
4. What a meal!

BBQ Steak/Chicken Wrap

Servings: 4
Calories: 405.5
Prep and Cooking Time: 00:20

Ingredients
8 ounces sliced - cooked steak/chicken breast
2 c baby spinach
4 (8-inch) whole wheat fat-free tortillas
1 c of each:
Frozen – thawed corn
Can black beans
½ c shredded cheese (low-fat cheddar)
¼ c barbecue sauce

Instructions
1. Rinse and drain the beans.
2. Program the oven temperature to 400F.
3. Lightly spray a baking dish. Roll up each of the wraps and
    heat thoroughly for ten minutes.

Chicken Philly Cheese Sub

Servings: 4
Calories: 409.0
Prep and Cooking Time: 00:40:00

Ingredients
1 pound chicken breasts
4 whole wheat hoagie rolls
4 slices provolone cheese
2 sliced bell peppers
1 sliced yellow onion
2 sliced banana peppers
¼ tsp black pepper
1 tbsp white wine vinegar

Instructions
1. Set the grill on the high setting. Flatten the meat with a mallet.
2. Grill the chicken for approximately ten minutes or until the internal temperature is at 165ºF. Let it cool a few minutes and chop into ½-inch cubes.
3. Coat a saute pan with non-stick cooking spray and add the onions. Saute for five minutes on the med-high setting.
4. Add the peppers and cook another ten minutes. Pour in the vinegar while scraping up the tasty bits and remove from the pan from the burner.
5. Divide the ingredients onto the buns, and top with a cheese slice. Wrap them in foil and grill two minutes so the cheese can melt.

Grilled Cheese Pizza Sandwich

Servings: 1
Calories: 242.3
Prep and Cooking Time: 00:30

Ingredients
2 tbsp marinara sauce
2 slices mixed grain bread
¼ c mozzarella cheese – part skim
Pepper and salt to taste
1 tsp shredded parmesan

Instructions
1. Divide the marinara sauce on each slice of bread.
2. Add the mozzarella to one with the sauce, parmesan, and add the second slice of bread.
3. Brown until the darkness you prefer.

Ranch Cheddar Turkey Burgers

Servings: 6
Calories: 155.1
Prep and Cooking Time: 00:25:00

Ingredients
1 (one-ounce) pouch dry ranch dressing mix
¼ c chopped scallion
1 pound lean ground turkey
1 c shredded cheese (low-fat)

Instructions
1. Mix all of the fixings and form six patties.
2. Cook on the grill/skillet about six to seven minutes for each side.
3. Enjoy with tomato and lettuce on a bun (not included in counts).

Tuna Salad

Ingredients
1 can tuna packed in water (6 ounces)
1 ½ tbsp mayonnaise
1 tbsp each:
Pickle juice
Powdered eggs

Instructions
1. Combine each of the ingredients in a blender or by hand until smooth.

Turkey Spinach Feta Burger

Servings: 6
Calories: 280
Prep and Cooking Time : 00:30

Ingredients

1 tbsp olive oil
20 ounces lean ground turkey
10 ounces frozen spinach
1 c diced red onion
2 minced garlic cloves
3 ½ ounces crumbled feta cheese
1 tbsp each:
Grilled steak seasoning (Mrs. Dash)
Chopped fresh oregano

Instructions

1. Thaw and drain the spinach – removing all water.
2. Saute the garlic and onion in oil, cool, and add to a dish with the oregano, and spinach. Blend in the feta, turkey, and seasoning to form six patties.
3. Cook on the grill/stove. Place on a bun if desired, but count the calories.

www.ingramcontent.com/pod-product-compliance
Lightning Source LLC
Chambersburg PA
CBHW062136020426
42335CB00013B/1233